WALL PILATES

for Seniors

MADE EASY

A **28 DAY STEP BY STEP** GUIDE TOWARD GREATER FUNCTIONAL STRENGTH, ENHANCED STABILITY, AND INCREASED VITALITY USING ILLUSTRATED EXERCISES

Brenda ten Bosch

Interior Design by FormattedBooks

CONTENTS

INTRODUCTION

*I*n the quiet cocoon of her 74 years, Ruth found herself standing on the precipice of change. Every day, she faced an internal uphill battle. It mirrored her external struggles as she tried to convince herself that change at her age was impossible. Ruth was unknowingly caught in a sedentary routine, as she found herself becoming more and more isolated. Ruth, like so many other seniors, used joint stiffness as a convenient excuse not to exercise. Depression lurked silently in the background. This exacerbated the sense of hopelessness she had to endure every day. Ruth was not aware of the fact that a lack of physical activity is yet another cause of mental health issues. So, she unknowingly continued on the downward trajectory of loneliness and depression, blaming the aches and pains in her joints as the perfect excuse for feeling "weak" due to old age. This is a common narrative amongst seniors.

Despite the obstacles, life still held potential. Ruth's revelation came in the form of a daily exercise routine. It was an intentional gift to her body that had faithfully supported her over the years. Making this choice was a powerful statement of resilience, given that she was now in the later stages of her life. Especially if exercise isn't part of your routine, as it was not part of Ruth's, deciding to revitalize your health and well-being at 74 requires a conscious mental shift to occur. It is important to make this shift by doing the exercises because this will restore your body to optimal health, regardless of your age. The idea is to take things one day at a time. You know already that your body at 74 is not identical to your 20-year-old self. However, you do not need to be discouraged by this. As long as you can move your body, it still presents an opportunity for exercise.

Wall Pilates serves as an excellent entry point for you to start cultivating a healthier lifestyle. It offers a more gentle approach to mobilizing your joints. I aim to guide you through an empowering, accessible, and manageable 28-day challenge. It is going to change your life. If you stick with this program, you'll soon find yourself on a trajectory of new growth, improved well-being, strength, and independence. These are the qualities that every senior deserves to experience. Exercise is a powerful tool, especially for seniors grappling with the psychological challenge of increasing dependence. So it is something to be excited about. Physical exercise can create a strong foundation for you to experience greater healing throughout your body, mind, and spirit. Beyond physical strength, exercising regularly sharpens the mind and rejuvenates the spirit.

Do stick with the program, to experience great results, and you can be the best judge of its effectiveness. Very soon you will be on the path to feeling good, strong, and independent. Celebrate that because even at 74, life is still a celebration. At the end of the 28-day challenge, the change will be obvious to you. You will feel elated with your progress, and following the hormonal release of dopamine, you will be happier than usual. Every senior deserves to enjoy vital health and wellness and to experience a sense of being in control of their ailments. When you engage in exercise, you will reclaim command over your body, sending a powerful message to your brain that improvement is your goal. The brain craves challenges, and your body yearns for both recognition and care, regardless of age. Exercise is not a form of punishment; it is a pathway to healing and self-recovery.

You have every right to savor life; it's your inherent birthright, and you deserve to live your best life at any age. Your body, too, deserves love and nurturing. If, like Ruth, you've been leading a sedentary lifestyle before discovering wall Pilates, her story stands as an inspiring testament of truth. In these pages, my mission is to persuade you why letting another day pass without exercise is not an option. It's the key to gaining strength, rekindling hope, and combating the decline in vitality that many seniors encounter. A remarkable revelation awaits you within the pages of this book. It is something you may have unintentionally overlooked, and I want to share this revelation with you right away.

Here it is: The key, when embarking on anything new, is to begin slowly and to treat yourself with gentleness. One of the most beautiful aspects of aging is the liberation you can experience from unnecessary ambition. Instead, we can slow down to embrace a gentle pace, which allows us to relish this state of flow, in each moment of our life. We can make exercise a vital part of that state of flow. It is about reclaiming vitality and bringing presence back into your life. The crucial step to initiate this process is to explore the myriad benefits of exercise, and we are going to do exactly that in this book. This is the ultimate gift you can give yourself, especially now in your senior years. Remember, every journey of a thousand miles commences with that very first step. I welcome you to this exciting journey of change, rejuvenation, and empowerment (Tweed, 2022).

The Stronger Person

Encouraged by both her daughter and her rheumatologist, Ruth embarked on her fitness journey, starting with physical therapy and later enrolling in a gym to explore the fundamentals of safe exercise. Her trainer introduced her to Pilates exercises that could be easily replicated at home. With an optimistic spirit, she thought, "Why not give it a try? The potential benefits seem promising, and what do I have to lose at this age?" It turned out to be a decision that significantly enhanced her life. Just as negative thoughts can easily creep in, Ruth discovered that she could just as effortlessly switch her mental gears to embrace positivity. This transformative mindset allowed her to live life one day at a time, fostering an outlook open to discoveries, even at the age of 74.

Ruth received invaluable advice from her rheumatologist. The same advice is offered to over 12 million American adults today, who are all grappling with inflammatory rheumatic diseases. Engaging in daily exercise not only alleviates joint pain but also mitigates symptoms associated with various diseases. This was the primary motivation behind Ruth's decision to give it a try. Her mild depression stemmed from the challenges of her condition and the accompanying pain. She was also lonely and isolated. Following her rheumatologist's advice, Ruth discovered that daily exercise increased muscle flexibility and positively impacted her mental well-being. Consider this: Depression often arises from overthinking, excessive worry, feelings of loneliness, or heartbreak.

It's not exclusively linked to a particular disease but can result from various mental health conditions or traumatic experiences. Those who've grappled with mental health issues or significant life transitions can attest that depression can stealthily manifest without warning. Medical health care practitioners consistently recommend daily exercise as an effective means of combating both anxiety and depression. Despite Ruth's initial skepticism and lingering belief that she might be too old and frail, she decided to heed the advice. She was also tired of living her life in a depressed mode. This choice, driven by her resilience and consistent inclination to take the less-traveled path, showcased her strength of character (*Exercise Can Help Patients with Rheumatic Disease Live Well*, 2013).

Choosing to engage in regular exercise is a wise decision. The advantages of exercise are universal, spanning across all age groups, but hold particular significance for older adults. For seniors, consistent physical activity plays a crucial role in easing joint discomfort and nurturing mental resilience. Anxiety and depression, often prevalent in older individuals, can find relief through a routine exercise regimen. Embracing this philosophy could serve as the linchpin for overcoming a myriad of challenges faced by seniors. If only a majority of seniors today embraced this approach, life might unfold as a smoother journey for them. This book is therefore tailored especially for those seniors who may be hesitant to commit to a daily exercise routine. If someone caring enough has gifted you this book, it's with the hope of lovingly persuading you to move forward and embrace vitality for yourself. It's never too late to reclaim inner joy for yourself.

Consistent exercise is the pathway to that rejuvenation, and it's a gift you can give to yourself each day. Numerous seniors who've already committed to my 28-day wall Pilates challenge have witnessed significant transformations in their health and well-being, and they continue to adhere to it. The majority of the seniors who have completed my 28-day challenge are now driven to sustain an active and healthy lifestyle in the long term. Even seniors without children are prioritizing health. Achieving and sustaining high levels of wellness remains a vital and compelling reason for them. Seniors who engage in regular exercise, especially those with children, aspire to cultivate enduring relationships with their children and grandchildren.

Their motivation is to have the energy and vitality to spend quality time with their children and grandchildren. They want to be fully present for them, and they desire to eagerly participate in the daily activities and priorities of their own life. Beyond external expectations, their internal motivation springs from an inner youthful well of inspiration—they yearn to feel capable and self-reliant. They want to bust the myths of old age and reclaim the spark of life that once animated their younger versions of themselves. Ruth encountered numerous challenges, throughout her new fitness journey. Initially plagued by self-doubt and the difficulty of adhering to a routine, Ruth contemplated quitting numerous times. Yet, the resilient and determined nature of her inner life propelled her forward, nudging her a bit further each day. Embracing self-compassion, she persevered through moments of wanting to quit, even if it meant sticking to the routine for just five minutes (Senior Tip, 2019).

You Got This!

As Ruth persisted each day with her brand-new exercise routine, the pull of negative thoughts weakened. She did her utmost best to ignore them and avoid the urge to quit. The more resilience she showed against negative urges, the greater her progress. Ruth found herself growing fitter, and her mind was also strengthening. Before she knew it, daily exercise, even if only for five minutes, became an ingrained habit. It's a well-known principle that if you stick to something for at least 21 days, it transforms into a habit. Ruth, however, discovered an additional layer: not only does a habit form after 21 days, but it also becomes challenging to break. Unbeknownst to her, the brain favors habits, and while forming new ones can be initially painful, they solidify over time. Ruth extended her commitment beyond the 21 days, understanding that habits, once ingrained, require less conscious effort. Initiating habits is a daunting process, as it involves unlearning old patterns and stepping out of one's comfort zone (Morero, 2022).

It's a mind-over-matter endeavor, similar to shifting the mindset from believing in weakness and incapability to embracing a new, empowering perspective. Shift the mind, and you will shift your life. Persistently adhering to her routine despite facing setbacks, Ruth began to observe subtle yet meaningful improvements in various aspects of her well-being. Enhancements in balance, flexibility, and strength became evident, marking positive progress. Additionally, she discovered a sense of community in the gym. Forging connections with fellow seniors, alleviated feelings of loneliness and isolation, ultimately boosting her morale. Motivated by these strides, Ruth extended her positive changes beyond the gym. Inspired by her progress, she adopted healthier food choices and became more socially engaged, shedding the cloak of solitude, isolation, and depression.

Choosing to reclaim your health and vitality brings forth an array of blessings. The key is patience, just as Ruth demonstrated to us in her resilience against negativity and in her gentle approach to her new routine. Taking things slow and gentle is an act of compassion, and it makes all the difference. Remember this as you begin your new inspiring journey. The rewards of your commitment and resilience will extend beyond the physical benefits that accompany daily exercise. Mental health and social improvements become integral aspects of the journey. This principle isn't exclusive to seniors; it resonates with anyone on the path of self-improvement. Daily exercise invariably reshapes how we think, feel, and experience life. Daily exercising fosters positive transformations that are accessible to everyone, regardless of age. It is my honor to guide you on this journey of physical transformation. Get ready to embrace the best version of yourself as a senior!

PILATES FOR THE GOLDEN YEARS

*D*espite his initial resistance, "back pain" prompted 72-year-old George to start wall Pilates. It is always a bit of a mental challenge to shift gears at first, especially when forming new habits. George was initially resistant because he was stuck in his ways. He enjoyed his routine. He was a prominent businessman and hall-of-fame Team Penning Cowboy. Let's just say George was always on the go. He led a busy lifestyle at 72 and had no appetite for changing anything in his current routine. Set in his ways, he wanted his life to stay exactly as it was. It wasn't that he shied away from physical activities. He enjoyed taking long trail rides in the countryside. However, he kind of frowned at stretching. It seemed like a slow, and tedious thing to do daily.

It was the urgency of his doctor's warnings and voice that made him pause to reconsider. So, George agreed to start with the basics to see how it went. "But no promises beyond that!" He insisted on this, as he beamed a smile at his trustworthy doctor. A promise was a promise, and being a gentleman of his word, George obliged and started doing some basic stretches daily. His doctor's advice resonated with George's age and physical condition. Stretching daily and exercising is the best advice that all doctors will offer to seniors. It makes perfect sense and aligns with the focus on senior well-being. Aging brings a natural slowdown to our lifestyle and activities.

Daily stretches can, however, shift the mindset completely, and as for your health, it is a powerful antidote to everyday challenges that accompany the aging process. Let's say (and it may resonate with you) that stretching is crucial to enhance joint movements and maintain flexibility. Activities like getting up from a chair become more challenging with age. The gradual decline in muscle strength and flexibility is a common aspect of aging. This is why Wall Pilates emphasizes the importance of flexibility for improved mobility. Any caring doctor for senior patients will stress the significance of daily stretching to facilitate better joint movement and overall well-being. It is a blessing, and once you get started you will experience a marked and positive difference on so many levels.

Positive Outcomes for Seniors

Everyone's fitness level and abilities are unique. Some of us already have unique health challenges as seniors that we need to accommodate. This is why it is so important to discuss your health issues with your medical doctor before you get started with Wall Pilates. You will receive great advice, just as George did. He was advised to stretch his arms, back, neck, legs, and hips. He needed a full-body stretch daily to keep himself limber, supple, and flexible. Many seniors don't know this, which is why it is worth mentioning over and over again—stretching prevents injuries and is *NOT* the cause of injuries. A study published in the Journal of Gerontology highlighted the positive outcomes of a 12-month flex program for seniors (Fruetal, 2016).

George is not alone in the troubles he has with his back. As you age, a common challenge is overcoming back pain. Because the emphasis is on core strength and achieving stability, it helps to alleviate back pain. Another result is an improvement in posture when actively participating in Pilates exercises and stretches. This reduces back pain. George noticed these improvements, and this is why his initial resistance to stretching daily faded away entirely. It felt good to walk straighter and feel strong from within without the familiar debilitating backache pulling him down. The daily stretching routine became a welcome part of his mornings, evolving into a daily habit that he looked forward to each day.

Surprisingly, integrating the daily stretching routine into George's busy schedule turned out to be much more manageable than he initially thought. Presently, George stands fitter than he was a year ago when he first started with his morning stretches, and he is so grateful that he switched his brain from thinking of it as a chore to a blessing. He completely attributes the positive transformation to his overall well-being to this newfound practice. It's time for you to experience similar benefits. Think of this shift in lifestyle as an affordable investment in a healthier, more active, and independent version of yourself.

Anticipate the rewards: enhanced freedom of movement, improved posture, and a boost in confidence—all contributing to an overall sense of well-being. Always remember that you are most deserving of this, and it is time to reward yourself with improved health and vitality. Think of your senior years as a fresh chance to radiate uniquely, to sparkle daily, and to honor your beautiful body for all the years it has given you. Seize the opportunity to live your best life every day.

The Genesis of Wall Pilates

Pilates has been around for 100 years. You'll be surprised to learn that cats played a prominent role in the history of Pilates. The story of Pilates began when a German trainer observed cats and how they appeared to be very agile and flexible. He also noticed that cats stretch a lot, and he attributed this to their flexibility. The German trainer went by the name of Joseph Pilates. He is largely credited with developing this type of exercise, which is best described as a series of controlled stretches. Joseph Pilates introduced this form of exercise in the early 20th century, and it gained immense popularity just after its debut introduction.

Over the years, Pilates evolved into a type of holistic healing system, since it is a combination of both physical and mental conditioning. Joseph was born in Germany, in 1883. A history of suffering from various health ailments, which included asthma, and rheumatic fever, made him very determined to prioritize health and wellness. This was his ultimate motivation for delving into various physical disciplines. Amongst his favorites were bodybuilding, martial arts, gymnastics, and yoga. It was this blend of physical activities that influenced the unique synthesis of exercises he developed. The discipline of his new exercise regimen would later become known as Pilates.

During World War I, his exercises became very relevant. While residing in England at the time, Joseph designed this new discipline of exercises to help bedridden soldiers rehabilitate. He attached springs to the beds of these bedridden soldiers to help them use a form of resistance when doing the exercises. When Joseph moved to the United States with his wife in 1926, they decided to set up an exercise studio. It was situated in New York City and his work attracted a diverse range of clients, such as dancers, athletes, and even more people who needed some kind of physical rehabilitation.

To this day, Pilates is still a popular exercise method. Its effectiveness lies in improving core strength, flexibility, and the overall well-being of those who engage in it regularly. Today, many fitness studios offer Pilates classes all over the world. It also continues to serve those who need rehabilitation. There are an estimated 12 million people who practice Pilates. People of all ages use Pilates for the same purpose that Joseph first developed the discipline: to strengthen their bodies, improve flexibility, and improve their overall wellness. In this way, Pilates is similar to yoga. For seniors, Wall Pilates is the best alternative to mainstream Pilates. It has only recently gained momentum as the ideal type for seniors (Nast, 2019).

Unpacking the Science of Pilates

There are plenty of reasons why Pilates is usually recommended as the best option for seniors to begin a physical exercise routine. We've encountered two remarkable narratives featuring Ruth and George, both showcasing how Wall Pilates positively influenced their health and overall well-being by overcoming resistance. Now, let's delve into the scientific rationale supporting the pivotal role of Pilates, especially for seniors. By unraveling these scientific foundations, we can better appreciate the holistic benefits that Pilates offers in enhancing physical health and fostering a positive state of well-being among older adults.

Low-Impact Nature

Firstly, Pilates is a low-impact physical activity. This means that it is a safe and joint-friendly exercise discipline. This is what makes it perfect for seniors. There's no hopping around or using equipment that could pose a danger to seniors. Pilates being low-impact makes a gentle and soothing way of taking care of both body and mind. Joint stiffness usually occurs when you suffer from conditions like arthritis. Doing Pilates means that you can still enjoy exercising without causing more pain to yourself. All the movements are controlled and there is an emphasis that is placed on achieving proper alignment. This by itself already reduces the risk that comes with impact-related injuries.

Core Strength and Stability

Pilates aims to improve core strength and stability for seniors. This is crucial to maintain good posture. The reason I am emphasizing achieving good posture is because it's important to acknowledge that as we age, maintaining a good posture can be challenging. Poor posture results in all sorts of health problems. Your spine is like a highway. When posture is correct, the nerves move down the spine to the muscles faster and more effectively. Good posture helps muscles move more appropriately. These include back pain, breathing difficulties, and neck pain.

Balance and Coordination

The movements of wall Pilates exercises are very controlled and well coordinated. This is important because it enhances neuromuscular coordination, which is also known as motor control. For seniors, this is important. As we age, our neuromuscular coordination declines. This can result in falls and other injuries. So, seniors need to do coordinated exercises that enhance motor control. In a study that was published by Life, it was noted that the physical endurance of older adults can improve by engaging in muscle training exercises (Concha-Cisternas et al., 2023).

Flexibility and Range of Motion

Another aging concern for seniors is the tendency for joints to lose their flexibility. This results in stiffness, which further impedes movement. Wall Pilates addresses these concerns. The carefully designed exercises engage various muscle groups in dynamic stretches. These movements increase the suppleness of the muscles and this in turn facilitates a much broader range of motion. For seniors, the benefits translate into increased flexibility and an overall improvement in functional movement. In this way, daily activities become manageable and enjoyable.

Mind-Body Connection

The movements that you will be engaging in are well-coordinated and very controlled. This results in creating mindful movements and hence wall Pilates promotes self-awareness, helping you to completely tune into your body. Gentle and effective exercises promote a state of mental calmness, which is a powerful cognitive tool. The result of strengthening a mind-body connection is helpful for seniors because it also enhances mental acuity (*Mind & Body Connection: Helping Seniors Stay Healthy - California Mobility*, 2019).

Safe and Adaptable

It is safe due to the support the wall offers during all exercises, and the exercises are very controlled. It is adaptable because anyone can adapt to the exercises easily. You do not need to achieve a certain level of fitness to enjoy the benefits associated with wall Pilates. All exercises can be modified to varying degrees of fitness levels. Adjustments can be made in a range of motions, intensity, and repetitions. The adaptable nature of wall Pilates therefore includes a gradual progression that is modified according to your fitness level.

Breathing Techniques

In Pilates, breathing is very important because this is how you will get the most out of your exercise routine. All low and high-impact exercises focus on breathwork. Pilates is an exercise discipline that relies on deep, controlled breathing. You will need to master your breathing to get the most out of your wall Pilates sessions. It is especially beneficial for seniors because it contributes to increased oxygenation. Remember to always breathe in through your nose, and out through your mouth. This is how you achieve deep breathing, which is beneficial when engaging in controlled movements (*Breathing in Pilates: Why It's Important | Pilates Principles | Club Pilates*, n.d.).

Stress Reduction

We all need an outlet to release stress. Your new wall Pilates sessions offer you the perfect chance to release a build-up of stressful energy in your body. All types of exercise afford us this benefit. Pilates is not an exception. You will feel so much better after a good stretch that incorporates mindful movements and deep, controlled breathing techniques. When you're fully present and engaging in physical activities, you will feel more optimistic and less bothered by trivialities. Pilates is calming by nature and therefore will contribute meaningfully to experiencing more tranquility (Menzies, 2019).

Improving the Quality of Your Senior Years with Pilates

Firstly, wall Pilates is a great full-body workout that is low-impact, versatile, and easy to fit into any schedule at home, at the office, or just about anywhere convenient. It is suitable for all fitness levels and is growing in popularity amongst all age groups, so it's not only for seniors. However, there are advantages for seniors to begin their Pilates journey this way. Firstly, it provides support and is a firm anchor for seniors with balance issues. If you're struggling with mobility or are concerned about being steady as you stretch, wall Pilates will remove that fear. It will give you immense confidence knowing that you won't have to worry about falling over or losing balance, which can be frustrating for a senior person. It, therefore, significantly reduces your chances of falling.

Additionally, Wall Pilates emphasizes the importance of achieving body alignment. The wall, therefore, serves as both a visual and physical guide for seniors. This is how it aids in improving posture throughout all exercises. In this way, it also improves bone density by adding tension to bones as you stand and balance. This is important for senior people. Wall Pilates can also be adapted to accommodate many different levels of fitness, as well as physical and health conditions. This is what makes wall Pilates accessible for seniors with diverse needs. Some exercises can be done standing only, if getting on the floor isn't an option. Ultimately, we can say with confidence that wall Pilates provides the perfect conditions for seniors to regain strength, flexibility, and posture and reduce pain in the back and joints. It is safe and fun and brings about a total transformation of body, mind, and spirit (Mazzo, 2023).

A Quick Recap of Main Points in This Chapter

Here's a quick summary of the main points of this chapter.

- Wall Pilates is safe for seniors and easy to fit into a daily schedule.
- It offers stability and significantly reduces fear associated with joint pain and falls.
- Wall Pilates is accessible and adaptable for all fitness levels.

- You can do this easily at home, as long as you have a safe space with a wall.
- Enjoy improved flexibility, significantly reduced joint pain and better posture.
- Say goodbye to the aches and pains associated with aging when doing simple tasks.
- You will feel more confident and walk taller!

Now that you understand the basics of wall Pilates and its importance in the life of a senior, it's time to kick-start our journey on the right foot!

STARTING OFF ON THE RIGHT FOOT

To embark on your wall Pilates journey, all you require is a compact, designated space in your home. Given that wall Pilates is executed using a wall, that's essentially all the space you need. Besides investing in a professional Pilates mat, no additional equipment is required. The practice of stretching in wall Pilates is inherently soothing. While the initial stages might present some challenges as your body acclimates to new exercises, adopting a gentle and paced approach is key. Take it day by day and treat each Pilates session as a deserved sanctuary for your body, mind, and spirit.

At the age of 68, Linda was introduced to wall Pilates by her physiotherapist. The journey began when she suffered an arm injury during a countryside holiday, which later evolved into a persistent disability. In her quest for a full recovery, Linda consulted a local physiotherapist named

Erin. To her relief, Erin assured her that the condition was treatable, not permanent. Filled with hope, Linda committed herself to following Erin's advice diligently. She was determined to heal and to use her arm again without experiencing pain. This was her primary motivation. It is important to come up with reasons to justify the new habit. It will fuel your action and produce great results.

Due to the mild to moderate nature of her arm injury, Linda was advised to incorporate daily gentle stretches into her routine. After a month of consistent stretching, Linda found herself inspired to take her routine to the next level by enlisting the help of a trainer. With her trainer's assistance, she established a dedicated wall Pilates space at home and quickly adopted a daily wall Pilates stretching regimen. This designated space helped her stay motivated and contributed to an increase in Linda's commitment and drive. Consequently, her daily exercise habits helped her achieve a complete range of motion in her arm. She was thoroughly satisfied with the positive results. Wall Pilates became an integral part of her daily self-care ritual.

Getting Started at Home

Consider Pilates not as a destination, but as a transformative journey. Your journey commences right here—X marks the spot. As you engage with this inspirational book, you're gearing up to focus on a 28-day challenge that has the power to revolutionize your life. Indeed, this is the commitment you're making. Whether it's striving for enhanced posture, increased mobility, flexibility, or mental and physical strength, the key is to persevere for 28 days with a positive mindset—even during challenging moments. This commitment proves to be a significant game-changer. The journey is liberating because consistent effort in anything new yields remarkable results. Each day dedicated to your

Pilates routine contributes to the continuous improvement of your overall well-being.

Taking small steps in a new direction maintains momentum, leading to wonderful changes in body, mind, and spirit. Once you've gone through this book at least once, the next step is to establish your own dedicated Pilates space at home. If you're truly committed and want to eliminate any excuses for missing a session, consider using a nearby gym or hiring a personal trainer for added motivation. However, for the present moment, let's focus on clearing a space at home, preferably next to a wall, where you can comfortably engage in stretching. Follow these steps to accomplish the second most crucial step in your new journey (Grebeniuk, 2022):

- **Designate a space:** The space you choose for your daily wall Pilates session should ideally be quiet and comfortable. It could be in your bedroom, study, or the corner space of your living room. Or you can choose to do it outside in your garden next to a wall. It is really up to you entirely.
- **Pilates mat:** Purchase a proper, professional, extra-thick Pilates mat that will support your spine. For extra comfort for your knees, glutes, or head, keep a cushion close by.
- **Comfortable clothing:** It is important to get the most out of your Pilates session, so choose loose, comfortable clothing that will not restrict you in any way whatsoever.
- **Pilates equipment (optional):** It is not necessary to invest right away in Pilates equipment, and you can go without it altogether. There is some optional equipment to purchase to complement your workouts. For example, small hand weights, a Pilates pad for neck support, or a mini resistance band for leg work might be good add-ons. You can also use a small hand towel rolled up to support the neck when lying on the floor.

- **Create a routine:** Plan your workouts by setting aside specific times of the day dedicated to Pilates. Sticking to a routine reinforces the habit, turning it into a lifestyle. This is what you should be aiming for.

- **Posture and alignment:** To avoid injuries and to get the most out of your Pilates exercise sessions, focus always on your posture, think about your movements, and aim to optimize the benefits by doing deep breathing exercises. Pause in between to think about each movement and pay attention to the alignment of your body during the stretches.

- **Warm-up and cool-down:** Make it a habit to never skip doing a small warm-up routine before jumping right in. Also, conclude your session with a cool-down. Warm-ups and cool-downs can further prevent injuries while improving flexibility.

- **Stay hydrated:** Keep a water bottle close by and remember to take generous sips in between each exercise.

Setting Yourself Up for Success

Let's approach this topic with honesty and sensitivity. Understandably, seniors may find it challenging to maintain the level of motivation they had in the past. Numerous factors contribute to this, with aging being a significant influencer. Personal factors can also play a role; emotional struggles and health concerns may make it easier for seniors to feel demotivated rather than inspired. Physical limitations further compound the issue, as they not only make daily activities more challenging but can also impact one's mental outlook. In some instances, the mind may reluctantly adapt to a slower pace of life, leading to a sense of defeat.

This emphasizes the importance of breaking free from any negative mental patterns. Constantly reminding yourself of the benefits that wall Pilates brings can be a powerful tool. Facing the daily challenge of accepting reduced strength, flexibility, and mobility can be mentally taxing. These physical limitations make certain activities more challenging, leading to frustration and hesitation. Hence, adhering to a simple and effective wall Pilates routine becomes even more crucial. Strengthening both your body and mind is essential to reclaiming independence. Aging is an inevitable aspect of life, and our choices and habits significantly shape the quality of our senior years. Consider how you want to live the next decade of your life. Don't give up movements that you want to keep for the future.

Overcoming the fear of injury is a significant hurdle for many seniors. This fear is especially real for those experiencing joint pains due to aging and a lack of regular stretching or exercise. Such concerns can weigh heavily on a person, causing them to question the value of engaging in an invigorating Wall Pilates routine. I consistently recommend that seniors address these worries by consulting a qualified medical professional— someone they trust. Speaking openly with a doctor can help alleviate fears, address concerns, and dispel doubts. It's in your best interest to reach out to a doctor, share your health issues, and seek guidance on approaching the 28-day challenge. For instance, if you're dealing with back pain, consulting with a doctor can provide assurance and guidance on the appropriateness of stretching exercises given your specific condition.

Seniors may encounter mental challenges that hinder their pursuit of adopting new healthy habits. These challenges are not exclusive to older individuals; even those who are young and fit can find mental health issues to be debilitating. Mental health struggles, including anxiety and depression, are not uncommon among seniors. According to the National Academy of Medicine, at least one in five seniors grapples with a mental health issue. The World Health Organization estimates that around 4% of seniors experience anxiety. For some seniors, anxiety is rooted in specific fears, such as the fear of falling due to poor balance. Interestingly, many seniors express greater concern about health issues compared to work or relationship issues (*Seven Common Mental Health Issues*, n.d.).

Beyond mental health issues, some seniors exhibit a fixed mindset. If you identify with this, transitioning to a more accepting mindset is entirely achievable. By engaging with this book, you're already taking the necessary steps to understand the significance of embracing wall Pilates as an important part of your lifestyle. Overcoming a rigid mindset involves empowering yourself with knowledge, dispelling aging-related myths, and cultivating a positive growth mindset that is receptive to change and adopting healthier habits and lifestyles. Setting a clear goal plays a pivotal role in motivation. You have the will to determine the quality of life, and remember, you are not alone on this transformative journey. Support is available when needed (Smith, 2022).

Tips for a Successful Pilates Practice for Seniors

To effectively address the challenges that may hinder your willingness to embrace change, it's essential to adopt a holistic approach. Here's what you can do right now to break free from resistance: Evaluate your physical, emotional, and social well-being to identify any sources of resistance to adopting a healthier and more active lifestyle. The next step is to recognize the interconnected nature of your thoughts and emotions. To achieve this, aim to scrutinize your mental state for negative thoughts, fears, or signs of anxiety and depression. Pilates, being a holistic approach to wellness, emphasizes the importance of mental well-being alongside physical health challenges. Consider these tips to help you maintain a successful Pilates practice.

- **Start slow**: Remember the story of the tortoise and the hare: A slow and steady approach will lead to your victory. Start with the basics and gradually increase your threshold for more intense exercises. In this way, your body can gently adapt to the new exercise routine.

- **Set goals**: Make sure that your goals are realistic and achievable. Whatever they may be, to increase flexibility, strengthen your muscles, or achieve overall wellness, write them down, then move in the direction of your goals.

- **Have fun**: You must have fun. Make it your special time to be one with body, mind, and spirit. Enjoy connecting to yourself in this manner. Find joy in each moment and use the breath of life to remind you how worthy you are of exercising and taking care of yourself.

- **Stay positive and don't give up**: Always keep your focus on the positive aspects of your progress. Approach challenges with a winning attitude. With persistence, you can overcome anything—so persist and keep moving forward, lovingly.

- **Consistency matters**: Your aim must be to ensure a consistent schedule with wall Pilates. Habits become a way of life when we remain consistent.

- **Don't be afraid to ask for help**: Ask for help if you need it instead of giving up altogether. There are lots of Pilates instructors now all over the world. So, wherever you are, look up a qualified instructor to get you started on the right foot.

- **Mix it up over the long term**: Keep yourself engaged productively by introducing other exercises and modifying your workout routine.

- **Keep it simple**: Focus on the simple techniques when you start. You will eventually master the basics and move on to higher levels of mastery.

- **Rest and recover**: Allowing your body time to rest and recover is important. Do this between sessions. Don't overdo it. Aim to keep up to a good, manageable pace. Get enough rest and reward yourself as you progress.

Core Pilates Principles

Joseph Pilates students created core principles to make his work more accessible to Pilates students. These core principles form the foundation of Pilates, and they help to guide people through a series of controlled movements that engage both the body and mind. Here are the core principles of Pilates (Smith, 2018):

- **Centering**: This principle revolves around engaging and stabilizing the core muscles. Specifically, the following muscles are engaged during a Pilates workout: the abdomen, hips, buttocks, and lower back. When you have a strong core, you will feel more centered and in control of your bodily movements.
- **Control**: All movements in Pilates are very controlled and precise. This is how you will be able to practice mindfulness while bringing your body into a state of flow while working out. The Pilates approach is focused on doing quality exercises as opposed to going for quantity.
- **Concentration**: All holistic practices that follow the path of the body-mind approach require concentration. This is how we connect mind to body and body to mind. When you focus on the movements, you will engage the muscles. This is how you can optimize your workout. The mind-body connection is a key element of Pilates. Go deep into it, immerse yourself in concentration, and enjoy each breath and movement.
- **Precision**: This refers to the movements you will be engaging in. Ensure that you are precise when moving your body. Each exercise is focused, precise, and targeted at certain muscles and areas of the body. Make sure that your movements are focused as you pay attention to alignment, posture, range of movement, and specific muscle engagements.

- **Breath**: Your breathing should be deep, as you connect body to mind and mind to body. Keep your breathing in rhythm with the flow of your movements. Joseph Pilates always strongly emphasized using the breath wisely to facilitate a wonderful flow state. Not only does it improve the oxygenation of your cells, but it also promotes deep relaxation. You will find that you will sleep better at night.

- **Flow**: The movements are designed to be graceful. As you practice Pilates, think of yourself as a graceful dancer. Move in a state of flow. Be fluid and unite with each movement. Your goal is to enter into a deep state of flow with your body. This is how Pilates enhances flexibility and improves your overall coordination of movement.

- **Posture**: Take a look at yourself as you engage in Pilates. What does your posture feel and look like? Are you comfortable doing the exercises? Pay attention to your posture throughout the session. Always aim for great posture. If it feels uncomfortable, look at your posture and choose to do a simpler move that supports your posture, instead of causing strain to any part of your body.

Common Pitfalls and How to Avoid Them

Before we move on to the next chapter, it is important to learn more about the common pitfalls when starting with Pilates. These are the typical mistakes we make as seniors when starting a new exercise routine. Now you can learn upfront how to avoid making the following mistakes and be on your way to a successful start on the right foot.

- **Overexertion (wrong intensity)**: Don't push yourself too hard. Relax and be gentle. Overexertion at anything, be it in sports or work, leads to fatigue and even burnout. When you overdo it, you also risk physical injury. You might experience sore muscles. Stop when this occurs and rest. Always start at a lower pace instead of moving to an advanced level too soon. You can always do more eventually, but you can't undo an injury.

- **Incorrect form**: Make sure that you do not overlook this aspect. It is important to get the alignment right from the get-go. When your posture is incorrect, you will add strain to your joints and muscles. Be gentle and kind to your body. You are doing yourself a big favor when you adjust your form and alignment to keep your posture strong.

- **Skipping the warm-up or cool-down**: Always do a warm-up and a cool-down before every workout. Warming up exercises increases the blood flow and prepares your body for the exercise. It also increases flexibility and reduces any risks of injury. The morning daily stretches are good to do as a warm-up. Cooling down prevents stiffness in the muscles and joints. Long, slow, lingering stretches are good for a cool down.

- **Ignoring pain, muscle imbalances, and nagging injuries**: Never ignore discomfort or pain, as it could lead to more serious problems. See to the pain immediately. Discuss it with a physiotherapist, doctor, or Pilates instructor and follow their professional advice. Slow down your sessions when you experience pain.

- **Rushing through movements**: Emphasize precision always. Avoid rushing through your exercises. Take your time, practice deep breathing, watch your alignment, and enjoy it. Be in the moment. Become mindful of your body-mind connection and enter a state of flow. Let go of any stress, worries, or negativity while exercising.

- **Forgetting to modify exercises**: We are all unique with individual challenges. Especially amongst seniors, it is necessary to modify the exercises as you go along. It is important to remember that modifying the exercises to suit what is manageable for you is not a sign of weakness. It is a smart approach. Improvement comes in phases, so be willing to walk your journey and modify where necessary. For example, if getting down on the floor is difficult, then start with the exercises that are standing only.

- **Skipping a rest day**: Listen to your body. You will have days that will require you to do no physical activity but just rest. Your body will remind you when it is most needed. Rest is an important part of the ongoing recovery process needed by your body. Overtraining can increase the risk of injuries. Do prioritize rest to allow your body to rejuvenate itself naturally.

A Quick Recap of Main Points in This Chapter

- In this chapter, we covered all the basics for getting started.
- Starting on the right foot means setting yourself up for success.
- It's to dedicate space at home for wall Pilates.
- Make sure you get an extra thick Pilates mat to support your spine.
- You deserve to achieve maximum results, so pay attention to your posture, movements, and breathing.
- Always strive to avoid injuries by being gentle and flowing into a routine without trying to achieve too much too fast.
- Have fun by making this your time to nurture and heal your body, mind, and spirit.

Your most important lesson as you begin this journey is to be patient with your body. Do not set unrealistic goals. You are doing this for you.

CHAPTER

3

YOUR CORE AND MORE

*E*velyn, a vibrant senior with a zest for life, remains determined to navigate the challenges that come with aging, even at the age of 72. Introduced to wall Pilates at her local community center, she embraced the idea of incorporating it into her daily routine. Since she was a little girl, Evelyn always loved trying new things. This is how she approached wall Pilates—with enthusiasm and curiosity. In her youth, she entertained a vivid imagination, always coming up with little adventures in the backyard of her family home. Playing alone was a source of joy. It allowed her to dive deep into her imagination. It made her feel liberated and independent. At 72, she still craves feeling liberated and independent. Wall Pilates gave her this chance to reclaim some of the lost vitality she experienced as she aged.

It was challenging at first. She most certainly wasn't a seven-year-old anymore playing in the backyard. She faced fears and encountered various new challenges. Her balance was unsteady, which caused her to fear stumbling with each step. However, she persisted and soon discovered a game-changer: the power of breath combined with wall Pilates. With a strong mind, she was determined to overcome the negativity associated with aging. Evelyn instinctively knew that she needed to move past her fears. She sensed more to discover on the other side of those fears. She began her wall Pilates journey and took her time to become familiar with each movement. Evelyn recognized the importance of mindful breathing as she progressed and began practicing it effectively before each Pilates session.

The wall became her reliable anchor during each suggestion, giving her confidence, especially considering her deep-set fear of stumbling. It granted her physical strength, and the wall removed her fears of falling. This support empowered Evelyn to master control over her movements. In a deliberate effort, she synchronized her actions with deep, intentional breaths—a practice that turned out to be the true game-changer. Deep breathing not only facilitated control but also played a vital role in dispelling the initial layers of anxiety that lingered within her. With a focus on her breath, Evelyn experienced a profound sense of peace. Standing firm and supportive, the wall evolved into a trusted companion throughout her journey.

Strengthened by its presence, Evelyn observed a noticeable transformation in herself, which she primarily attributes to the transformative influence of deep breathing. This newfound harmony with breath enabled her to enter a flow state, marking a significant milestone in her wall Pilates journey. The rhythmic inhales and exhales heightened her mindfulness, creating a profound connection between her body and mind. In those moments, she experienced a heightened sense of presence. Once merely a support, the wall assumed a new role in her practice. Over time, she developed increased confidence in aligning her movements with her breath, transforming the wall from a crutch into a canvas for her graceful motions.

Evelyn discovered the significance of deep breathing during her Pilates workout. Deep breathing provided comfort, alleviated anxiety, stress, and fears, and helped her enter a flow state by connecting with her movements. Moreover, it induced deep relaxation and improved sleep. At the end of each day, she was grateful for her Pilates session. It brought her rest and tranquility. This state of joy put her in touch with her inner life. In wall Pilates, the importance of proper breathing cannot be overstated. It has a profound impact on wellness. Breathing serves as a link between movement and relaxation during a Pilates session, fostering mindfulness and presence.

Evelyn experienced this firsthand during her wall Pilates session. Breathing is not just a static element but a dynamic and crucial aspect. Its healing nature extends beyond its physiological functions, acting as a bridge between movement and relaxation. Effective breathing cultivates a stronger mind-body connection, enriching the holistic approach to wellness and physical health in Pilates. Let's explore how breathing transforms the overall Pilates experience in more detail (Sharder, 2021).

- **Connection with movement**: As already discussed, breathing in Pilates is not just physiological; it is part of the holistic journey of improving mindfulness. Breathing mindfully will harmonize your movements while bringing a sense of calm and rejuvenation at the same time. Keep your movement graceful, and let it be guided by your breath—the breath of life and vitality. Every inhale and exhale is a cue to a movement. In that way, it is similar to yoga. Inhales and exhales become cues for movement. This synergy ensures a deeper connection between the body and the mind.

- **Mind-body harmony**: Conscious and coordinated breathing during Pilates helps to achieve that ecstatic state of body-mind harmony. Directing the breath to your movement creates a heightened self-awareness, increasing presence and leading to mindfulness. Think of the breath as the guiding force to a higher state of consciousness while removing the layers of distracting thought. Anything you're focussing on with precision and deliberate intent is bound to increase presence. In Pilates, the breath focus increases mindfulness and helps participants concentrate on achieving good alignment and strong movements.

- **Relaxation and stress reduction**: In Pilates, mastering effective breathing techniques not only contributes to relaxation but also provides significant stress reduction benefits. Deep breathing activates the body's parasympathetic nervous system—also known as the rest and digest mode. The more consistently you practice deep breathing, the more profound your ability to combat stress and anxiety becomes.

- **Physical responses to deep breathing**: As you engage in deep breathing, your heart rate gradually slows down. It extends to the muscles and promotes overall relaxation. This practice not only enhances your physical well-being but also sharpens your mental focus. By cultivating mindfulness through deep breathing, you become more anchored in the present moment, fostering a sense of attentiveness. This "presence" contributes to an overall reduction in stress and anxiety levels.

- **Improved oxygenation**: For seniors, prioritizing deep breathing is pivotal. This practice enhances the body's oxygenation levels, a critical factor for optimal well-being. Elevating oxygenation contributes to improved functioning of vital organs and plays a central role in achieving overall health and wellness. Specifically, the benefits of enhanced oxygenation extend to the cardiovascular system, strengthening the heart's ability to circulate oxygen-rich blood throughout the body.

- **Core engagement**: Breathing also provides a foundation for core engagement in Pilates. When there is a good flow and coordination of breathing and movement, the effectiveness of each movement improves. The more you practice deep breathing during your exercise sessions, the greater your chances of strengthening core muscles. A strong core aids in achieving functional effectiveness in everyday living because a strong core brings these benefits: improved balance, stability, less risk of falling, reduction in back and joint pain, improved posture, and support to internal organs (Blanchfield, 2022).

The Pilates Breathing Method (Lateral Thoracic Breathing)

The Pilates breathing method forms a core part of the Pilates practice. To maximize the impact of your daily wall Pilates routine, it is important to understand how it works so that it becomes a practical part of your ongoing Pilates discipline. Using this breathing method as much as possible during your movements will contribute to a deeper sense of holistic wellness. I invite you to explore a detailed explanation below (Blanchfield, 2022):

- **Thoracic expansion:** This refers to the lateral expansion of the thoracic cage, involving the ribcage as well as the intercostal muscles. The idea is to breathe deeply into the sides and back of the ribcage. Avoid shallow breathing, by connecting to the ribcage.
- **Diaphragmatic engagement:** Lateral thoracic breathing involves engaging the diaphragm. When you inhale deeply, the diaphragm contracts and moves downward. This allows the lungs to expand and maximize the intake of oxygen.

- **Enhanced core activation:** Lateral thoracic breathing is an integral part of engaging the deep stabilizing muscles of the core area. When you breathe deeply in this manner, you will enhance the activation of the transverse abdominis. This is how you can provide ongoing support to your spine.

Common Breathing Mistakes

As you've just learned, breathing is pivotal to any Pilates practice. You need to be aware of certain common mistakes as they can hinder the effectiveness of your Pilates sessions. When done incorrectly, breathing may lead to discomfort or even injury. Here are some breathing mistakes that seniors might make when practicing wall Pilates (*Here's What You're Doing Wrong...*, 2023).

Mistake	Impact
Shallow breathing	It limits the oxygenation levels in your body, resulting in fatigue, exhaustion, and diminished overall performance.
Holding your breath	Avoid holding your breath. It is unhealthy to do so. It increases tension in your body and your mind and limits the flow of oxygen to your muscles. It can also elevate blood pressure.
Irregular breathing patterns	This refers to what is known as erratic breathing. It usually disrupts the flow of movements.

Rapid or slow breathing	Rapid breathing may result in hyperventilation and anxiety. Slow breathing may reduce oxygen levels in your blood.
Breathing in the chest	Breathing only from the chest reduces the amount of oxygen in your body.
Ignoring exhalation	This is a common mistake for most people. By not giving proper focus to exhalation, you will create tension in your body. It can also result in ineffective movements.
Breathing through the mouth	You will lose control over your breath this way. It may also result in a dry mouth.
Lack of mindful breathing	When you fail to pay attention to your breath, you can feel a diminished sense of connection between body and mind.

Tips to Correct Breathing Mistakes

- **Focus on diaphragmatic breathing**: This is the correct way to practice deep breathing. The emphasis is on the sides and back of your ribcage.
- **Establish a smooth pattern**: Get into a steady rhythm for inhalation and exhalation. Work it in such a way that it complements your movements.

- **Practice mindful breathing**: Always stay attentive to your breathing. This is how you will achieve more mindfulness during each Pilates session.
- **Incorporate nasal breathing**: Incorporate more of this and consciously exhale through your mouth. This is how you will optimize the wellness of your entire respiratory system.

It is important to be conscious of common mistakes. Now and then during the day, pause to reflect on your breathing and to rectify any mistakes you're making (*Deep Breathing Exercises, Benefits and How to Breathe Correctly*, 2013).

A Breathing Exercise: The Diaphragmatic Breathing Exercise

If you perform this regularly for at least five to ten minutes, you will gradually take to it more naturally. Do this, especially before each Pilates session. It is especially beneficial for seniors, and it will assist you in creating a more mindful way of breathing. This type of breathing will also increase your level of focus. It also optimizes the functioning of your lungs. The focus is on the diaphragm (Manheim, 2023).

Follow These Steps Before Each Pilates Session

- **Get into a comfortable position**: Sit comfortably on a chair or the floor. As long as you're comfortable. You may also lie down on your Pilates mat. Keep one hand on your chest and the other on your abdomen.
- **Relax completely**: Check to see if there's any tension in your body. Release that tension and adjust and relax by preparing to focus singularly on your breathing.

- **Inhale through the nose**: Inhale deeply. Keep your inhalation slow, deliberate, and deep. Pay attention to your abdomen. Feel it expand as you fill your lungs with oxygen.
- **Exhale:** Exhale slowly through your mouth. Take your time. Enjoy the feeling of a gradual contraction of your diaphragm as you gently release the breath.
- **Continuously repeat the breathing pattern:** Keep going with this rhythmic breathing. If you can help it, do it consciously many times throughout the day, and you will undoubtedly experience a marked difference in wellness.
- **Increase the duration if necessary:** As you become more comfortable with this deep diaphragmic breathing, increase the duration. You can also use this method during meditation, to maintain a centered, and calm state of being.

Posture and Alignment

It was Oscar Wilde who famously said that with age comes wisdom. However, he did not live long enough to reap the benefits of aging. He died at the age of 46. Often, as seniors, we get beset by so many issues, which we need to pause to reflect on the blessings of aging. We've lived a long life, and we still have the golden years to enjoy (even though the journey seems rather short upon reflection). If you are mindful of what you are facing health-wise, nothing is stopping you from still going for your dreams. We go through life with multiple identities from the moment we are born. In our senior years, we adopt a new identity. This is why sometimes it can be mentally taxing to make new adjustments to an aging body. It is how you adapt and take control of the aging process that counts. Your mental attitude will ultimately determine your true state of happiness and the choices you make for your health.

One of the most fundamental changes we go through is watching a decline in our posture. It's a fact that we can no longer stand up as straight as we once did. That's because the spine weakens as we age. It may become more curved. Spines have a natural curve, but aging wears it down over time. A big contributing factor is persistent neck and back pain throughout the years. The most affected part is between your neck and lower back. This part is known as hyperkyphosis. It is also known as "hunchback." The implications for seniors with this condition of the back can be as follows: reduced mobility, risk of falls, pain, discomfort, and impaired breathing, which can result in lung problems. Here are some of the factors that contribute to this condition known as hyperkyphosis (Cristol, 2021):

- **Muscle weakness**: Aging results in a decline in muscle strength. Those muscles that support the spine weaken over time and contribute to a more curved back.
- **Bone density**: Osteoporosis is a condition that is caused by lower bone density. It is a common condition for seniors, and this also increases the chances of hyperkyphosis developing.
- **Discs and joints**: Over time and with aging, the discs and joints of the spine change, and this may result in the development of hyperkyphosis.
- **Sedentary lifestyle**: Hyperkyphosis can develop if you are not getting enough movement. Sitting for long periods is a contributing factor. So, move more and more. Wall Pilates sessions in the day are exactly what you need to get some movement into your lifestyle.
- **Genetics**: This too plays a role in your chances of experiencing hyperkyphosis. It is in your genes. Some people are more prone to this due to their genetic disposition.
- **Changes in connective tissues**: These changes impact the ligaments and tendons, which further impacts the flexibility of the spine.

Preventing the Severe Impact of Spine Issues

There are things you can start doing today to take proactive steps to prevent the development of hyperkyphosis. It also comes down to having a positive attitude, as opposed to accepting a situation that may feel beyond your control. There are strategies that you can implement into your lifestyle from today to reduce your chances of hyperkyphosis developing:

- **Good posture**: Do this consciously whether you're sitting or standing. Keep your chest lifted, back straight, and aligned well. Do avoid slouching or hunching over.
- **Regular exercise**: Stick to a solid exercise routine that emphasizes the muscles of the back and core. The top choices to achieve this are Pilates and yoga, as these exercises specifically target the upper back.
- **Core muscles**: When you focus on strengthening the core muscles, it will give more stability to the spine. This is what supports proper alignment.
- **Thoracic extension exercises**: Choose exercises that encourage thoracic extension. You will find these in your wall Pilates sessions. The movements help counteract the curvature of the upper spine.
- **Body mechanics**: Give attention to your body mechanics throughout the day. When you lift objects, bend at the hips and knees instead of rounding the spine. Also, avoid lifting heavy objects as much as possible.
- **Balance and stability exercises**: Choose exercises that improve your balance and stability. This is how you can prevent falls and reduce the risk of injuries that cause hyperkyphosis.
- **Healthy bone density**: Ensure you get adequate calcium and vitamin D to support bone health. Engaging in regular

weight-bearing exercises, such as walking or some lightweight training. This, too, can help maintain healthy bone density. You can incorporate light weights into your Pilates session.

- **Don't sit for too long**: Do some stretching or go for a walk to break up long sessions of sitting for many hours. You can also make use of ergonomic furniture to ensure that your posture is not being compromised. Your body is made to move.
- **Health check-ups**: Get regular health check-ups. An early detection of any health issues can prevent further harm if treated accordingly.
- **Consistency**: Be consistent in your efforts to reduce the risk of injury and practice regular wall Pilates sessions.

When you follow the above strategies, you increase your chances of maintaining good posture and reducing the risks of developing hyperkyphosis. Always consult with a healthcare professional for personalized guidance.

A Quick Recap of Main Points in This Chapter

- Be vigilant of your breathing habits.
- Aim to breathe deeply from your diaphragm.
- Take your time before each Pilates session to practice deep breathing.
- Get into a regular daily practice of mindful breathing.
- Avoid shallow breathing and the list of breathing mistakes cited in this chapter.
- Maintaining good posture is an everyday challenge for seniors.

Begin your journey today by embracing these fundamental techniques to elevate your Pilates practice and improve both your physical strength and mental well-being.

SAFE AND SOUND

*I*n the quietude of her living room, Pam eagerly embraced daily wall Pilates sessions. It was her way of reclaiming vitality. Armed with determination, Pam diligently took her position next to the wall. She was very eager to advance and always pushed herself. The exercises are gentle, so when you push yourself too hard, there is a risk involved, as Pam soon discovered. The idea is to be gentle and let your body guide you to a comfortable limit. With any program, it is essential to listen to your body, take appropriate cues from it, and seek enjoyment as you gradually increase your fitness level. Generally speaking, people of all ages must follow this advice. Overdoing it and not listening to your body can result in injury and burnout. Your body needs time to adapt to the new routine, and so does your mind.

When you push yourself beyond your limits, you signal to your mind that you're in a rush to get results. Don't be hard on yourself. This is a demotivating factor from a mental health perspective. Therefore, aim to avoid it. From a physical perspective, you are moving away from the Pilates philosophy of promoting holistic healing and wellness. The aim is to be gentle, listen to your body, and get into a comfortable rhythmic flow, regardless of your fitness level. Pilates promotes mindful living. Therefore, you must be attuned to your body's needs and limitations. Keep this in mind as you begin your journey: Developing a strong connection between your mind and body can be achieved by tuning in to your body.

This is how you can obtain and maximize the beneficial effects of exercise on both your physical and mental health. There is no shortcut to success, not even with Pilates. So, ease into it. Pam suffered an injury early on because she failed to adhere to this important philosophy. Be enthusiastic in a way that is supportive and not unrealistic. See Pilates as a new way of life that must be gently worked into your routine, guided by your body's ability to adjust naturally. Pam was enthusiastic, but she was unrealistic. She was captivated by the movements. However, in her eagerness to master each pose, she neglected the core principles of wall Pilates. As enthusiasm took the reins, the subtle cues of mindful breathing and respecting personal limits slipped through the cracks.

Pam pressed herself against the wall hard, attempting to achieve a deeper stretch. But she soon discovered that she must pause to listen and feel her way through her body's signals. The wall is meant to be a supportive ally. You won't enter a graceful flow state with the wall if you push yourself too hard. You might find yourself fighting against it. Pam tossed the rules of Pilates out the window, and she became competitive, completely ignoring the principles of controlled movements associated with Pilates. In this way, she rushed through the exercises. She was driven by a strong desire to excel rather than to nurture herself.

I hope this will not be your encounter as you earnestly begin your journey. Take it one step at a time and don't push yourself too hard.

Rather, it is tiny steps that you take as you allow your body to guide you gracefully. You are not going into battle. If you find yourself becoming competitive or overestimating how fast you can improve, remember these words: You are taking this journey with serenity, love, and appreciation for the years your body has given to you. Honor it, be gentle, and don't be concerned about any other goal, but to get the movements right, watch your posture, be graceful, breathe deeply, and stick to a consistent routine that incorporates rest days in between. It was only when Pam healed from the injury she sustained as she pulled a muscle while stretching, that she started to appreciate the principles of Pilates. She then understood that it underpinned the effectiveness of Pilates for seniors (*Nine Facts You Should Know...*, n.d.).

You see, all wall Pilates isn't just about the movements. It is about the journey you're taking to integrate physical and mental well-being.

Recognizing Your Boundaries

The essence of fulfilling and sustainable practice lies in understanding and respecting your physical limits. Guided by the lessons she learned, Pam delved into the essential principles of Pilates once more to ensure that she properly integrated them into her movements. She also practiced deep breathing more frequently throughout the day, even as she enjoyed walking out in nature. Mindful breathing and mindful movements soon became the cornerstone of all her daily activities. She immersed herself in the present moment, and this further strengthened the holistic nature of Pilates for her. Remember that you aim to forge a positively inspiring and harmonious relationship with your body, mind, and spirit.

It is time to highlight more benefits of identifying and respecting your physical limits. Allow Pam's experience to serve as a poignant reminder.

As you approach each Pilates movement introduced in this book, treat each movement as an opportunity for a deeper connection and dialogue with your body. I also encourage you to embrace each movement as a wonderful celebration of your unique journey. Let's explore the key things that will improve the safety of your Pilates journey. While we do so, think of safety, mindfulness, and physical well-being as the three pillars supporting Pilates's effectiveness.

- **Your body sends signals:** Your body communicates with you through sensations. These are the signals you need to look out for. Ask yourself, where is there discomfort as you work out? If you're experiencing pain, then stop at once, or you risk more serious injury. The sensations are indicators of your body's limits. The threshold will improve over time, so be gentle.

- **Pay attention:** Deepen your awareness of your body's limitations. Always pay attention to what feels comfortable and what does not feel comfortable. In this way, you will be cultivating a mindful awareness of what is safe for you. Be fully present for each movement. Allow yourself to experience the sensations your body emits during each movement. Ask yourself: Does it feel comfortable, is it enjoyable, etc.? Explore them.

- **It's a skill to listen to your body:** Always aspire to listen to your body. It takes practice to become fully in tune with your body, but it's achievable. Engage in dialogue with your body when you eat, sleep, relax, and attend to your daily chores. In this way, listening to your body will soon become a skill to be proud of. Remember that your body is always communicating with you. You just need to tune into that dialogue. Understand the language your body speaks during Pilates movements.

- **Set realistic expectations:** Pam was unrealistic in her expectations, even though her motivation was high. It is important to set realistic goals. Don't beat yourself up if you are conservative.

It is better to be safe than to be injured. Therefore, see yourself realistically and consider your body's will to move and adjust. Allow it to guide you. Know your fitness level and health challenges before commencing your Pilates journey.

- **Do not compare yourself with others:** Be mindful of your unique journey. We are all unique, and you are not lacking in any way just because you're a beginner. We are all beginners now and then. Even accomplished athletes must return to basics after taking a long break from their grueling physical workout routine.

- **Follow natural movements:** You know your body always communicates with you. Allow it to guide you in your physical goals. Follow its cue and allow it to lead the way forward. Don't force your body into difficult positions. It must feel comfortable, natural, and flowing. Work with your body and treat it as your best friend. Go with its natural rhythms and flow.

- **Always proceed with caution:** This applies to you, especially if you're a beginner to wall Pilates. Take it easy and proceed with caution. This is sound advice. Introduce each of the movements gradually. Practice the ones that are new first to get the movement right before moving on to more advanced movements.

- **Pain and discomfort:** When there is pain, stop immediately. Rest your body until the pain subsides. Avoid becoming disillusioned by pain. It's a sensation that is saying somehow you pushed it too much for today, it's time to rest and heal. Discomfort is also a signal to pause or stop. It may also be related to a more difficult movement. If this is the case, don't do this movement or do an easier version of it.

- **Loss of form:** If your movements are no longer graceful and controlled, causing incorrect posture, it is a signal to pause. You may be tired or need to go back to learn how to achieve alignment with a particular movement. Alignment is a crucial factor when it comes to preventing injuries.

- **Breathlessness:** Take a break if you feel light-headed or breathless. You might need to stop altogether and rest your body before restarting Pilates. You should also assess the level and intensity of your workouts to bring them down a notch.
- **Persistent discomfort:** This is your cue to shift your movements to adjust better. Avoid pushing through the discomfort. It would also be best to avoid seeking guidance from a Pilates instructor.

By applying these careful and important considerations, you will empower your Pilates workout and feel strong, in control, and mindful of your ongoing choices. Pilates is a unique journey of deepening a more holistic approach to self-discovery. To achieve growth, vitality, and well-being, you must nurture this journey every step with positivity, encouragement, patience, diligence, and gentleness (*Pilates Safety: Minimizing Risks and Preventing Injuries*, 2023).

Preventing Pilates Injuries

As your journey begins, prioritizing safety should be a paramount foundational goal. Get it right from the start to avoid becoming demotivated by the lack of care taken on your part to prevent injuries. When we suffer from any injuries related to our efforts to improve health and physical form, it brings us down. Don't let this happen to you, so take the best care by following all the advice offered in this chapter to ensure your safety. This section will explore how to prevent "common injuries." They usually take the form of muscle strains, ligament sprains, and "Delayed Onset Muscle Soreness (DOMS)." Pilates is safe, but like any workout, it can cause injury if done incorrectly. This section discusses five common Pilates injuries and how to avoid them (*Pilates Safety: Minimizing Risks and Preventing Injuries*, 2023).

Neck Strain

This is a typical Pilates injury, but it is easy to avoid. Pay attention to how you control your neck during movements. The idea is to keep it neutral and to use your core muscles to support your head and shoulders. Keep your neck neutral and do not put any pressure on it when raising your legs, for example. If your neck hurts or feels uncomfortable during a movement, then stop immediately. Neck pain is also extremely common when you get started. You can also place your head down on a pillow to relax the neck in between exercises. Once your core is strengthened, you will feel the activation in your core muscles (*What to Do If You Have Neck Pain in Pilates*, 2023).

Lower Back Pain

Once again, you risk injury when you don't adequately support your lower back. This injury is common, especially for seniors. Even when lifting heavy objects, you must activate your core muscles, not your lower back, as you risk injury. Keep this in mind because it is important regarding the strain you may put on your lower back: Seniors above 50 are vulnerable to lower back injuries (Ullrich, 2019). This is due to the wear and tear that occurs over the years to your spinal structure. You must take care when you bend or twist during workouts. Do so gently and activate your core muscles. Also, watch your alignment and posture. Bend your knees slightly when bending. Stop immediately if you experience pain in your lower back.

Knee Pain

Improper knee alignment when you bend or twist can result in knee pain. By keeping the knees in line with your toes, you will engage the core to support the legs. This is the best way to avoid knee pain. Arthritis is another cause of knee pain. You can modify the exercises to avoid knee pain. This is an important reason for consulting with a Pilates instructor and a medical professional to discuss your physical ailments before commencing this journey. In that way, they can advise you on how to avoid certain exercises that may put more pressure on the knees. Stop the workout and adapt if your knees hurt (*Pilates and Knee Pain: Understanding the Causes and Solutions*, 2024).

Shoulder Pain

Improper form or shoulder support during Pilates results in shoulder pain. Once again, engaging the core and maintaining good alignment during exercise can prevent shoulder issues. If your shoulder pain is caused by an earlier injury or strain, consult with a Pilates instructor or a medical expert to gain more perspective. There are specific exercises you can do in this case to reduce inflammation and pain. However, if your shoulders hurt during a workout, you can modify the exercise or avoid doing overhead exercises where shoulder movements are involved (Menzies, 2021).

Wrist Strain

Wrist strain may occur when your wrist is not properly supported during hand-bearing movements. This is why it is important to distribute the weight evenly across both hands. Engage your core muscles to support your wrists. This will prevent wrist strain. Alternatively, you can modify the exercises or stop exerting your wrists by avoiding those exercises that are putting pressure on your wrists. A good modification is using your forearms instead of your wrists by resting on your forearms instead of applying pressure to the wrists. You can also rest between exercises to reduce any pain or pressure that you may be experiencing (*Pilates Tips and Modifications for Wrist Pain*, n.d.).

Tailoring Pilates to Your Health

Always remember that modifying an exercise to suit your health is not a setback but a strategic choice. It is encouraged that you do this. We are all unique with health challenges that we understand at an individual level. It is more than okay and perfectly acceptable to adapt your exercises to suit what your body can handle. As you progress, it is encouraged that you continue to listen to your body to gauge how far you can advance in your routine. Additionally, be sure to seek guidance from a qualified Pilates instructor or healthcare professional to guarantee an experience that is both effective and enjoyable, tailored to your specific needs. Let's embark on an empowering journey exploring modifications of wall Pilates for seniors. Keep the following considerations in mind as you customize Pilates to best align with your health. (Bartlett, 2018):

- **Avoid feeling shame when modifying:** Do not hesitate when modifying. It is necessary to tailor wall Pilates exercises to suit your needs.
- **It does not mean that you're cheating in any way:** You must dispel any notion that associates modification with cheating. It is there to make your life easier so you will not be deprived of exercise.
- **You will enjoy more control of the muscles and joints when you modify:** This is a fact. It also helps to foster more comfort and enjoyment.
- **You will still reap the benefits:** You will achieve all the associated benefits of doing wall Pilates regardless of modifications.
- **Effectiveness is enhanced:** When you modify, you increase the effectiveness of the movements while minimizing risks and associated injuries.

- **Modifying doesn't mean easy:** It does not mean that modification results in Pilates becoming easier than usual. It brings more comfort and increases safety.
- **There is no such thing as modifying too much:** Modify as much as is necessary to make the journey comfortable by the needs and recommendations based on your body's limitations and physical issues.
- **Respect the natural pace of your body:** Always listen to your body and respect its pace and flow. Your modifications must align with the needs and sensations of your body.
- **Consult with an instructor and health care professional:** Always do this if you're experiencing pain or discomfort, and it is advisable to do this at the outset before you begin this journey.

A Quick Recap of Main Points in This Chapter

- Make safety a priority when exercising.
- Remember to listen to your body by paying attention to any sensations that emerge during your workout.
- Pain and discomfort are important signals from the body to modify your exercises or stop altogether.
- We have discussed the most common injuries incurred during Pilates in this chapter.
- Prevention is better than rushing through an exercise without following the principles of Pilates: Be gentle, practice mindfulness, watch your alignment, and be careful about overdoing it.

The importance of safety, personalization, and professional advice in Pilates, should not be overlooked. Take them seriously.

Make a Difference with Your Review by Unlocking the Power of Hope

Dear Friends!

Have you ever discovered something wonderful—like a simple, effective exercise routine…or a stretch that makes your body feel better—and felt compelled to share it with others?

In the same way, that's the beauty of leaving a review.

It's more than just giving your opinion; it's about extending a helping hand to someone who is struggling and needs a little encouragement to move forward.

When you share how this book has helped you, whether it's easing into movements that felt impossible or finding joy in daily routines, you help illuminate the path for others. It's about solidarity, showing that change is possible and beneficial at any age.

Why Your Reviews Are Important

Your words have the power to uplift spirits and illuminate the bright possibilities that await in the golden years. You're not merely sharing your story—you're bestowing hope and courage on someone else, empowering them to embark on their own transformative journey.

How to leave your mark...share your experience by leaving a review!

You don't need to write much—just a few sincere sentences. What truly matters are your honest thoughts and heartfelt reflections. Consider the parts of the book that inspired you to take action and share those moments with others. That's it!

Writing a review is easy, and it means so much! Here's how you can help:

1. Go to the place where you bought "Wall Pilates for Seniors Made Easy."
2. Find the page for our book.
3. Look for the part that says 'Customer Reviews' and then click on 'Write a Review.'
4. Tell everyone about what you liked best. Which moves do you enjoy? How has the book made your days better?

Or, just use this QR Code and it will take you to the page on Amazon

I am deeply grateful for the time you're dedicating to help enrich the lives of others by leaving a review. Your effort truly means the world to me.

Thank you deeply,
Brenda

STRETCH, STRENGTHEN, AND BALANCE

*J*oe is a spirited 67-year-old who has defied the conventional notion of aging. He is a very active senior. He can often be spotted on his bike exploring scenic routes. He is passionate about cycling and fitness, and he is a source of inspiration to other seniors in his neighborhood. However, despite his enthusiasm for fitness, one of his biggest challenges for a long time was doing standing exercises. You see, balance issues have been a source of irritation for him for many years following a cycling accident. He sustained some knee injuries, and ever since, he's struggled with balance. He paid a price for his passion for cycling. It is not uncommon for cyclists to suffer from leg injuries. However, at his age, it was bothersome to him, and quite rightfully so, because balance issues are a major cause of falls.

In 2015, a study published in the "Aging and Disease Journal" delved into the prevalence of dizzy spells and imbalance among US seniors, particularly those over 72. The findings revealed that approximately 24% of seniors in this age group experience these issues, posing a significant concern due to the deep-seated fear of losing balance (Austrew, 2022). This worrisome statistic underscores the importance of addressing balance concerns among seniors. Fortunately, there are proactive steps individuals can take to enhance their balance over the long term. With consistent effort, one can mitigate the fear associated with balance issues. However, the effectiveness of the action plan hinges on identifying the root cause and making a comprehensive medical check-up imperative.

Joe's experience serves as a case in point. For him, the key to improving balance is strengthening his leg muscles. Pilates emerged as an effective solution, especially for individuals dealing with balance issues stemming from past physical injuries or weakened muscles. By tailoring the approach to address the specific cause, individuals can take targeted steps to regain balance and alleviate associated fears. Joe consulted with a medical expert to understand his balancing issues and to get right to work on correcting them. The tips he received included exercises to build strength in his legs. He wanted to feel more stable and not risk another cycling injury.

By embarking on daily stretches and standing leg exercises, he committed himself to achieving a specific goal, and with consistency, Joe achieved a remarkable transformation which included a newfound confidence. Joe's story is a testament to the remarkable achievements that unfold when one approaches a goal with unwavering determination. When you consistently practice wall Pilates, you will gain strength, balance, and confidence, which will positively impact all areas of your life. Now that you understand the philosophy and principles behind wall Pilates and how it will benefit you daily, it's time to begin the journey.

Part A

Morning Stretch Exercises

Now, let's jump right into your daily wall Pilates routine. Begin by dedicating 15 minutes to daily stretches—it's an invigorating start! As you embark on this for the first time, mentally commit yourself to making it a part of your daily routine. Starting your day this way is not only exciting, but also incredibly encouraging. Perform each of the stretches listed below five times. After finishing the first set, proceed to repeat the exercises for a second set. This completes your 15-minute daily stretching routine.

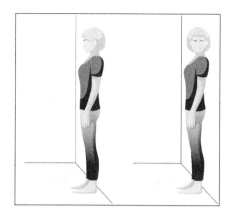

Neck Stretch Side-to-Side

- The first step is to stand up straight with your back against the wall.
- Keep your shoulders, arms, and hips against the wall.
- Keep your head pushed back against the wall.
- Keep your chin parallel to the floor.
- Both arms are placed straight to your sides.
- Turn your head to one side.
- Hold for five to ten counts.
- Now move your head back to the center.
- When you are ready, turn your head to the other side.
- Hold for five to ten counts.
- Repeat this for at least five times.

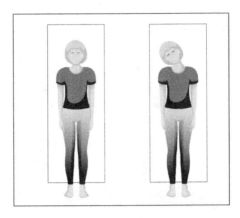

Standing Neck Stretch Ear to Shoulder

Once again, you will begin in the usual standing position as follows:

- The first step is to stand up straight with your back against the wall.
- Keep your shoulders, arms, and hips against the wall.
- Keep your head pushed back against the wall.
- Keep your chin parallel to the floor.
- Both arms are placed straight to your sides.
- Nod your right ear to the right shoulder.
- Hold for five to ten counts.
- Now move your head back to the center.
- When you are ready, nod your left ear to your left shoulder.
- Hold for five to ten counts.
- Repeat this for at least five times.

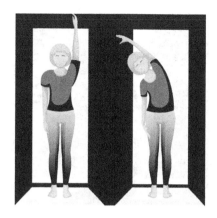

Standing Side Bends

Once again, you will begin in the usual standing position as follows:

- The first step is to stand up straight with your back against the wall.
- Keep your shoulders, arms, and hips against the wall.
- Keep your head pushed back against the wall.
- Keep your chin parallel to the floor.
- Both arms are placed straight to your sides.
- Bend your knees slightly into a 1/4 squat position.
- Keep your abs tight.
- Inhale and exhale deeply a few times.
- When you're ready to raise one arm, let's start with the right arm.
- Next, gently bend your arm and your right side for a stretch.
- Reach to the side until you feel a stretch.
- Be sure not to overstretch your side, it must feel comfortable but effective at the same time.
- Repeat this stretch with the other side and hold for five to ten counts.
- Now do these stretches at least five times on each side.

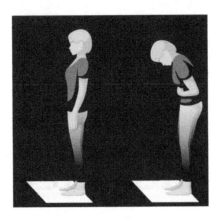

Standing Forward Folds

Once again, you will begin in the usual standing position as follows:

- Stand up straight with your back against the wall.
- Keep your shoulders, arms, and hips against the wall.
- Keep your head pushed back against the wall.
- Keep your chin parallel to the floor.
- Keep your feet a few inches apart and feel comfortable.
- Both arms are placed straight to your sides.
- Relax and inhale through your nose.
- Exhale through your mouth.
- Keep your abs tight.
- Gently roll down your upper body to fold over slightly.
- Make sure that your lower body is comfortable and strong.
- As you roll forward, move one vertebra at a time off the wall.
- Push your hips back and reach a halfway down position.
- Stop when you reach your hips.
- Hold here for five to ten counts.
- Feel the stretch and enjoy it while doing deep breathing.
- When you're ready, roll back up gently, one vertebra at a time.
- When you reach a standing position, take a few deep breaths.
- Do this stretch at least five times.

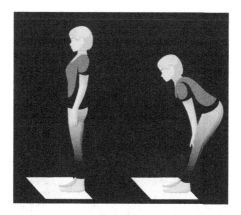

Standing Forward Hip Hinge

Once again, you will begin in the usual standing position as follows:

- The first step is to stand up straight with your back against the wall.
- Keep your shoulders, arms, and hips against the wall.
- Keep your head pushed back against the wall.
- Keep your chin parallel to the floor.
- Both arms are placed straight to your sides.
- Relax and inhale through your nose.
- Exhale through your mouth.
- When you're ready, move your feet at least 12 inches away from the wall.
- You will need to hinge forward at the hip to lengthen your back without bending your back.
- They should be in front of you.
- Hold it here for 10 counts.
- Remember to take deep breaths.
- Make sure that your back is lengthened.
- Your hips are pressed into the wall.
- Keep both legs straight.
- When you're ready, hinge gently, extending the spine.
- You are moving your arms forward at the same time.
- Place your hands on each knee.
- You are now stretching forward at your hips.
- Repeat this stretch for five times.
- Remember to inhale and exhale deeply as you bend forward over your hips.

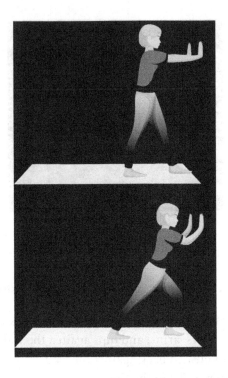

Standing Forward Calf Stretch

- You will change your standing position for this stretch.
- Stand up straight facing the wall.
- Make sure to inhale deeply through your nose and exhale through your mouth.
- Keep your arms straight and relaxed.
- When you're ready, bend your left knee at the knee and move it forward.
- Keep your right leg stretched behind the left knee and at an angle.
- As you move into this stretch, place both palms of your hands on the wall.
- Use the wall as a source of resistance for the stretch.
- Hold this position for at least five to ten counts.
- Then move back into your standing position facing the wall.
- When you're ready, repeat this on the other side.
- Repeat this stretch five times on each side.
- Remember to inhale and exhale deeply as you stretch your calves.

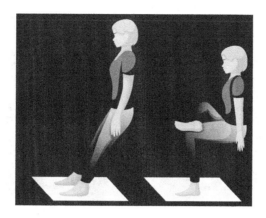

Four Stretch Standing

- Stand with your back leaning against the wall but keep your legs slightly apart and slanted (at a 45-degree angle) in front of you so that only your buttocks are against the wall.
- Make sure to inhale deeply through your nose and exhale through your mouth.
- Keep your arms straight and relaxed.
- When you're ready, raise one leg over the other while moving into a 1/4 squat position.
- Your right foot should be placed on one knee. It's as if you are sitting on a chair with your buttocks against the wall and one foot firmly on the ground.
- Hold this position for five to ten counts and enjoy the stretch.
- When you're ready, repeat this on the other side.
- Repeat this stretch five times on each side.

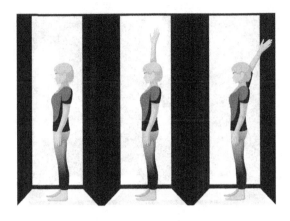

Side Facing Arm Circle

- Stand sideways, with either the right or left side facing the wall.
- Make sure to inhale deeply through your nose and exhale through your mouth.
- Keep your arms straight and relaxed.
- Raise the arm that is against the wall straight in front and above your head, keeping your hand on the wall at all times if possible.
- Once your arm is above your head, make sure that your palm is facing the wall.
- Press the wall if necessary, and gently lean away from the wall to allow a range of motion; don't force or strain.
- Hold the wall by placing the palm of your raised arm against the wall.
- When you're ready, turn your body in the opposite direction to repeat this stretch with your other arm.
- Do not strain, you may have to move away from the wall a little to keep connected to it.
- Repeat the exercise three times on each side.

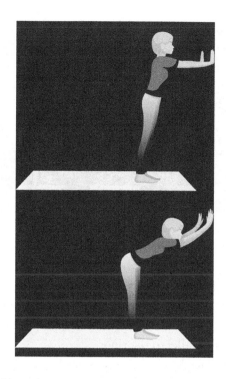

Standing Full Reach Lat Stretch

- Stand up straight facing the wall.
- Relax and inhale through your nose.
- Exhale through your mouth.
- When you're ready, place the palms of both hands firmly on the wall and slightly wide apart from each other.
- Stand at a slight angle with both legs straight.
- Do not bend at the knees.
- When you're ready, lean the hips back.
- Drop your chest toward the floor.
- Keep both hands straight as you press them into the wall.
- Hold this position for five to ten counts.
- Repeat this stretch for five times.

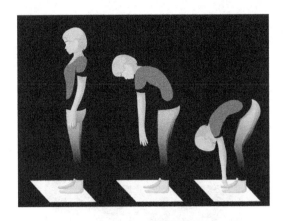

Standing to Roll down

- Stand up straight with your back against the wall.
- Keep your shoulders, arms, and hips against the wall.
- Keep your head pushed back against the wall.
- Keep your chin parallel to the floor.
- Both arms are placed straight to your sides.
- Relax and inhale through your nose.
- Exhale through your mouth.
- When you're ready, slowly round your back forward, starting from the neck.
- Then gently nod your head down.
- Then roll your upper back, and lower back forward as you reach your entire upper body, including your arms, towards your feet.
- Keep your knees slightly bent as you move down.
- Hold this stretch for five to ten counts.
- Then slowly reverse the roll by moving your body gently back upwards.
- Keep the movement deliberately slow by moving it one vertebra at a time.
- Keep rolling up gently until your spine is alright and you are back in the standing position when you started.
- Repeat this stretch five times.

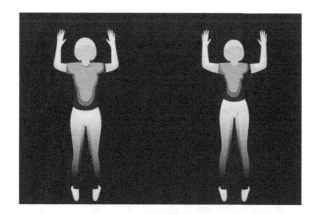

Standing Corner Chest Stretch

- This exercise is done in a corner of the wall.
- Each arm is placed on different walls as you gently lean into the corner.
- Raise the forearms on each side, placing the palms of your hands on the wall with shoulders down.
- Stand up straight, while keeping your feet firmly planted on the ground, slightly apart and comfortable.
- Relax and inhale through your nose.
- Exhale through your mouth.
- Press forward with your palms and hold this stretch for five to ten counts.
- Repeat this five times.

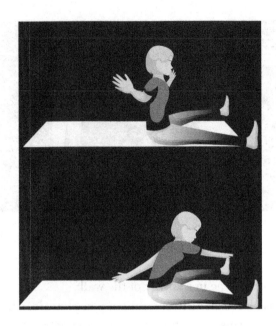

Seated Straddle Twist "Saw"

- Sit up tall on the floor.
- Keep your upper body erect and forearms outstretched at shoulder height.
- Your legs must be wide apart and your feet against the wall.
- Relax and inhale through your nose.
- Exhale through your mouth.
- When you're ready, move one arm behind you and the opposite one to reach the opposite foot.
- If your left arm is behind you, then your right arm will lengthen to touch your left foot or calf but don't strain.
- You are gently twisting to reach your opposite foot with one arm.
- Hold this stretch for five to ten counts.
- Repeat five times.

Part B

Standing Leg Exercises (Weeks 1, 2, 3, and 4)

When it gets difficult to do simple movements like standing or getting up from a chair or in and out of bed, then that is a direct cause of declining muscle flexibility. When you stretch your legs daily you can lengthen and stretch your leg muscles which will improve movement in the joints (Freutel, 2016).

Leg Exercises for Weeks 1 and 3

The following standing leg exercises should be done during weeks 1 and 3. Make sure to do three sets of five to ten repetitions on each leg.

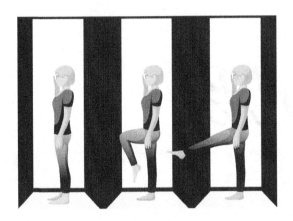

Standing Knee Lifts

- Stand straight with one side facing the wall.
- Raise the forearm facing the wall so that the palm of that hand is placed on the wall.
- Touch the wall lightly.
- Relax and inhale through your nose.
- Exhale through your mouth.
- When you're ready, raise the opposite leg to knee height.
- The leg that you are raising is the outer leg.
- Bend the knee of the outer leg toward the chest.
- Hold it here for three to five counts.
- Next, extend the leg in front before placing it down.
- Repeat this five times on each side.

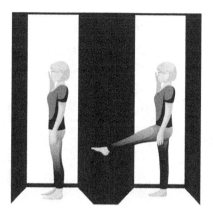

Standing Leg Lifts

- Stand straight with one side facing the wall.
- Raise the forearm facing the wall so that the palm of that hand is placed on the wall.
- Touch the wall lightly.
- Relax and inhale through your nose.
- Exhale through your mouth.
- Keep your abs tight.
- Make sure that you are standing tall.
- When you're ready, lift your outer leg straight up in front of you.
- Hold for three counts.
- Then gently return it to the ground.
- Make sure that you are not swinging your legs up and down.
- Keep the stretch controlled and focused.
- Watch your posture.
- Repeat this five times on each side.

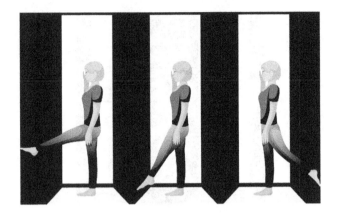

Standing Leg Circles

- Stand straight with one side facing the wall.
- Raise the forearm facing the wall so that the palm of that hand is placed on the wall.
- Touch the wall lightly.
- Relax and inhale through your nose.
- Exhale through your mouth.
- When you're ready, raise your outer leg gently forward.
- Then slowly circle to the side, and toward the back, and then return to a stand.
- Repeat this five times on each side.

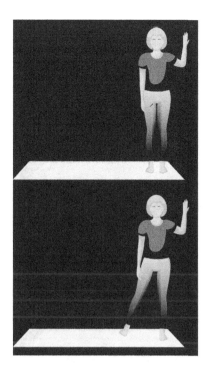

Standing Leg Side Lifts

- Stand to face one side of the wall.
- Place your forearm against the wall lightly.
- Make sure that you are standing tall.
- Keep your abs tight.
- Relax and inhale through your nose.
- Exhale through your mouth.
- When you're ready, raise the outer leg to the side gently, and then return it in place next to the other leg.
- Focus on leading with the heel.
- Do not swing or bend at the knees.
- Keep your movement controlled, smooth, and flowing.
- Repeat this five times on each side.

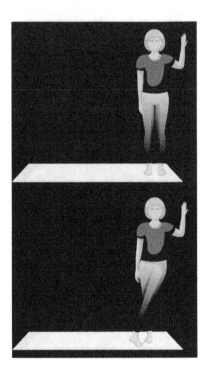

Standing Leg Inner Thighs

- Stand to face one side of the wall.
- Place your forearm against the wall lightly.
- Make sure that you are standing tall.
- Keep your abs tight.
- Relax and inhale through your nose.
- Exhale through your mouth.
- When you're ready, lift the inner leg, slightly across to the other leg toward the outside.
- Focus on lifting with the heel.
- Your legs should be crossed at the knees but do not bend the knees.
- Hold this stretch for three to five counts.
- Repeat on both sides five times.

Exercises to Cover for Weeks 2 and 4

The following standing leg exercises should be done during weeks 2 and 4. Make sure to do three sets of five to ten repetitions on each leg.

Standing Leg Hip Extensions

- Use your entire body to face the wall.
- Lean directly into the wall using your entire body.
- Keep your hands stretched out straight in front of you, with palms placed firmly and flat on the surface of the wall.
- Slightly bend your right leg at the knee and raise it behind you for a stretch.
- Make sure you are not swinging the leg.
- Raise it only a quarter of the way for a stretch.
- Relax and inhale through your nose.
- Exhale through your mouth.
- Hold for five to ten counts.
- Then gently return the leg.
- Repeat on the other leg.
- Do this strengthening exercise five times on each side.

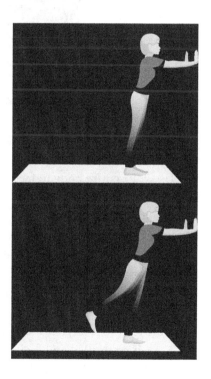

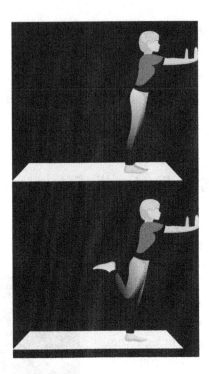

Standing Leg Curls

- Use your entire body to face the wall.
- Lean directly into the wall using your entire body.
- Keep your hands stretched out straight in front of you, with palms placed firmly and flat on the surface of the wall.
- Slightly bend your right leg at the knee and raise the calf upwards for a stretch.
- Keep your foot flexed and not pointed.
- Make sure you are not swinging the leg upwards at the knee.
- Curl your foot to your buttocks, then slowly lower it.
- Keep it controlled and focused.
- Relax and inhale through your nose.
- Exhale through your mouth.
- Hold for five to ten counts.
- Then gently return the leg.
- Repeat on the other leg.
- Do this exercise five times on each side.
- It can also be used to strengthen your legs.

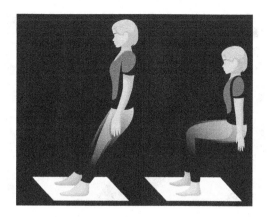

Standing Wall Squats

- Keep your back firmly against the wall.
- Your feet should be about 12 inches away from the wall.
- Stand with your arms tight.
- Slowly lower your body down the wall as if sitting in a chair.
- Relax and inhale through your nose.
- Exhale through your mouth.
- Be careful to not be on a slippery surface.
- Only go as low as possible.
- It would help if you did not experience any pain or discomfort in your knees.
- Hold for five to ten counts.
- Then gently raise your body again.
- Take a few deep breaths before repeating for five times.

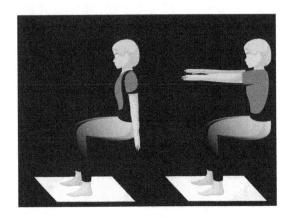

Standing Wall Squats with Arm Reaches

- Keep your back firmly against the wall.
- Your feet should be about 12 inches away from the wall.
- Stand with your arms tight.
- Keep your abs tight.
- Slowly lower your body down the wall as if sitting in a chair and pushing your back against the wall with strong tension.
- Relax and inhale through your nose.
- Exhale through your mouth.
- Be careful not to be on a slippery surface.
- Only go as low as you can.
- It would help if you did not experience any pain or discomfort in your knees.
- Raise both arms straight in front of you, keeping them at shoulder length.
- Hold for five to ten counts.
- Then raise them wide to the wall, and slowly return down toward the side.
- Then gently raise your body again straight up.
- Take a few deep breaths before repeating this strength exercise five times.

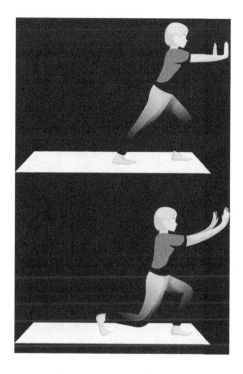

Standing Lunges Toward the Wall

- Lean directly into the wall using your entire body.
- Keep your hands stretched out straight in front of you, with palms placed firmly and flat on the surface of the wall.
- Bend your right leg at the knee and lower the left knee toward the ground. Only go as far as it is pain-free.
- Do not keep your left knee on the ground.
- Only go as far as you can get up.
- It would help if you were standing with your legs in a lunge position.
- Remember not to go too deep if you are experiencing pain in your knees.
- Keep it controlled and focused.
- Relax and inhale through your nose.
- Exhale through your mouth.
- Hold for three to five counts.
- Then gently return the leg.
- Repeat on the other leg.
- Do this strength exercise five times on each side.

Part C

Floor Leg Exercises (Weeks 1, 2, 3, and 4)

Stronger legs mean that you will overall improve your mobility, and you will be able to include some type of cardio training exercises into your daily routine. You also lower the risk of injuries when you strengthen your legs. Please note that if you cannot get down on the floor, then you can do variations on the bed (Woods, 2020).

Exercises to Cover for Weeks 1 and 3

Do the following exercises during weeks 1 and 3 on the floor using your legs. Do three sets on each side, repeating each exercise for five to ten sets.

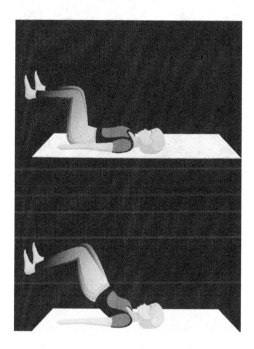

Bridges on the Wall

- Lie down facing up.
- Bend your legs at the knees with your feet firmly planted on the wall.
- Your feet should be kept at hip-width apart.
- Knees bent at a 90-degree angle.
- Raise your hips in the air.
- Contract your glutes as you do this.
- Your arms should be straight and flat on the floor.
- Keep it controlled and focused.
- Relax and inhale through your nose.
- Exhale through your mouth.
- Hold for five to ten counts.
- Repeat five times.

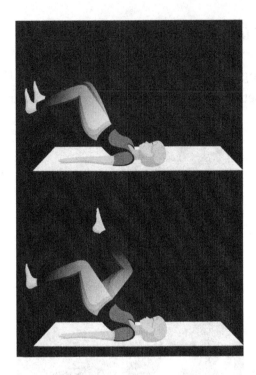

Bridges With Marches

- Lie down facing up.
- Bend your legs at the knees with your feet firmly planted on the wall.
- Your feet should be kept at hip-width apart.
- Knees bent at a 90-degree angle.
- Raise your hips in the air.
- Contract your glutes as you do this.
- Your arms should be straight and flat on the floor.
- Then lift one leg to your chest, and keep the hips up if possible.
- Alternate the legs and keep the movement controlled.
- Also, keep the spine neutral and the core engaged.
- Relax and inhale through your nose.
- Exhale through your mouth.
- Repeat five times on each leg.

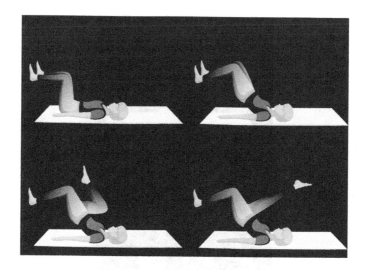

Bicycle Bridges on the Wall

- Lie down facing up.
- Bend your legs at the knees with your feet firmly planted on the wall.
- Bend one knee toward the chest.
- Then lift it toward the ceiling.
- Return leg to bent knee position.
- Make a cycle-like motion, then switch legs.
- Your feet should be kept hip-width apart.
- Knees bent at a 90-degree angle.
- Raise your hips in the air as you raise each leg.
- Contract your glutes as you do this.
- Your arms should be straight and flat on the floor.
- Alternate the legs and keep the movement controlled.
- Also, keep the spine neutral and the core engaged.
- Relax and inhale through your nose.
- Exhale through your mouth.
- Repeat five times on each leg.

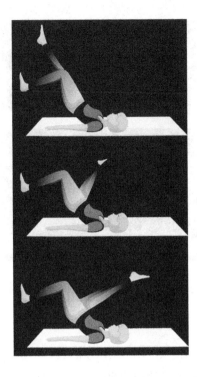

Bridges With Leg Circles

- Lie down facing up.
- Bend your legs at the knees with your feet firmly planted on the wall.
- Your feet should be kept hip-width apart.
- Knees bent at a 90-degree angle.
- Raise your hips in the air as you raise each leg.
- Contract your glutes as you do this.
- Raise one foot and straighten the leg straight up toward the sky.
- Then make a full circle with that leg.
- Return leg to bent knee position.
- Switch legs.
- Keep the movements controlled.
- Also, keep the spine neutral and the core engaged.
- Relax and inhale through your nose.
- Exhale through your mouth.
- Repeat five times on each leg.

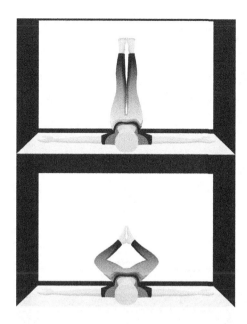

Wall Frogs

- Lie down face up.
- Keep your hips against the wall as close as you can manage.
- Extend your legs straight up and against the wall.
- Keep your arms stretched wide and horizontally flat on the floor.
- Then lower both feet so that they touch each other in a frog position.
- Relax and inhale through your nose.
- Exhale through your mouth.
- Repeat five times and hold for five to ten counts.

Exercises to Cover for Weeks 2 and 4

Do the following exercises during weeks 2 and 4 on the floor using your legs. Do three sets on each side, repeating each exercise five to ten times.

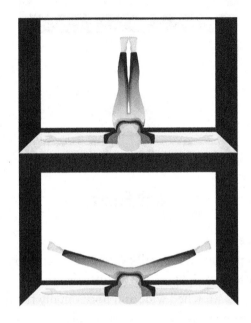

Wall Splits

- Lie down face up.
- Keep your hips against the wall as close as you can manage.
- Extend your legs straight up and against the wall.
- Keep your arms stretched wide and horizontally flat on the floor.
- Open your legs wide apart but gently without bending at the knees.
- Stretch the legs into a split.
- Then slowly return to the start position while pressing heels into the wall.
- Engage the core throughout the movement.
- Relax and inhale through your nose.
- Exhale through your mouth.
- Repeat five times and hold for five to ten counts.

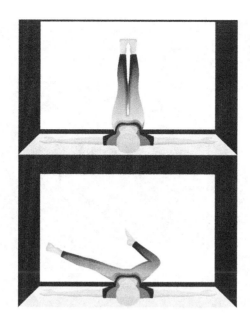

Wall Peter Pan

- Lie down face up.
- Keep your hips against the wall as close as you can manage.
- Extend your legs straight up and against the wall.
- Keep your arms stretched wide and horizontally flat on the floor.
- Bend one leg like a frog.
- Keep the other stretched straight out to a side split.
- Then bring both legs together again.
- Switch to the opposite side in the same manner.
- Engage the core throughout the movement.
- Relax and inhale through your nose.
- Exhale through your mouth.
- Repeat five times and hold for five to ten counts.

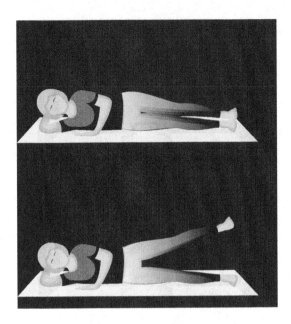

Wall Side Lying Leg Lifts

- Lie down on one side.
- Keep your body against the wall.
- Engage your core for this stretch.
- Leave one hand underneath your head (the bottom arm).
- Legs should be placed straight on top of each other.
- Inhale and exhale deeply.
- When you're ready, lift the top leg up and down the wall, pressing your heel against the wall throughout the movement.
- Your foot must be flexed as you move the leg for 30 seconds.
- Then repeat with a pointed foot.
- Hold for three to five counts before you lower the leg.
- Repeat this five times.

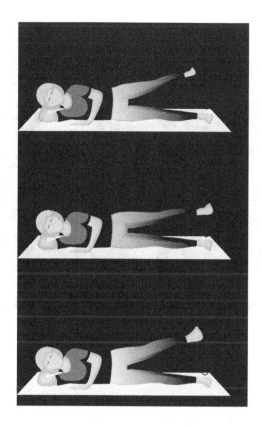

Wall Side Lying Leg Circles

- Lie down on one side.
- Keep your body against the wall.
- Engage your core for this stretch.
- Leave one hand underneath your head (the bottom arm).
- Legs should be placed straight on top of each other.
- Inhale and exhale deeply.
- When you're ready, lift the top leg about hip height.
- Make small six-inch circles with legs fully extended for 30 seconds.
- Repeat this three times on each leg.
- You would need to change your position to ensure that the bottom leg will now be on top.

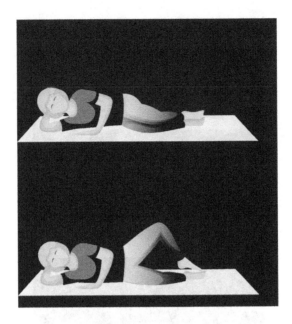

Wall Side Lying Clams

- Lie down on one side.
- Keep your body against the wall.
- Engage your core for this stretch.
- Keep one hand underneath your head (the bottom arm).
- Lift the top leg at the knee up and down without letting the hip move forward while pressing your heels together lightly.
- Inhale and exhale deeply.
- When you're ready, lift the top leg about hip height and squeeze tight for three counts, then slow release.
- Then lower the leg.
- Repeat this five times on each leg.

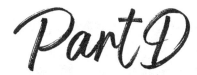

Part D

Standing Arm Exercises (Weeks 1, 2, 3, and 4)

Arm stretches to increase flexibility and range of motion in each arm. For seniors, it's important to keep your arms stretched regularly. It also helps to maintain good posture and functionality.

Functional Strength in the Upper Body

Regular arm stretching can also help with any stiffness you may be experiencing in your shoulder. Think of the different functions you use your arm daily like reaching to grab something from a high shelf, or microwave (*Arm Stretches for Seniors and the Elderly*, n.d.).

Exercises to Cover for Week 1 and 3

Do the following arm strength exercises during weeks 1 and 3. Do three sets of five to ten repetitions.

Standing Wall Push-Ups Wide

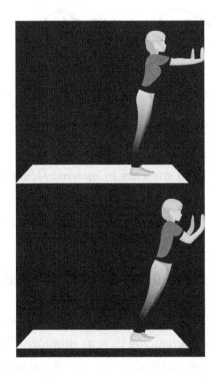

- Lean directly into the wall using your entire body.
- Keep your hands stretched out straight in front of you, with palms placed firmly and flat on the surface of the wall.
- Keep both legs straight but at a slight angle.
- Your arms should be straightened when you start.
- Remember to keep your movements controlled and focused.
- Relax and inhale through your nose.
- Exhale through your mouth.
- When you're ready, push against the wall by bending your elbows as you do that and leaning more inwards on the wall.
- Slowly lower your chest toward the wall, bending your arms back wide, then squeeze your chest as you extend your arms.
- Hold for three to five counts.
- Then repeat for five sets.

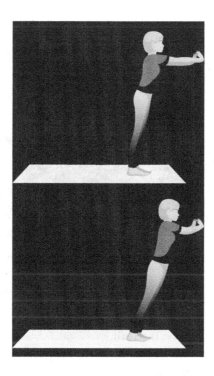

Standing Wall Push-Ups Narrow for Triceps

- Lean directly into the wall using your entire body.
- Keep your hands stretched out straight in front of you, with palms placed firmly and flat on the wall's surface.
- However, make sure they are close together, narrowed with palms closer together.
- Keep both legs straight but at a slight angle.
- Your arms should be straightened when you start.
- Remember to keep your movements controlled and focused.
- Relax and inhale through your nose.
- Exhale through your mouth.
- When you're ready, push against the wall by bending your elbows as you do that and leaning more inwards on the wall.
- Slowly lower chest toward the wall, bending arms back, narrow against the side of ribs.
- Hold for three to five counts.
- Then repeat for five sets.

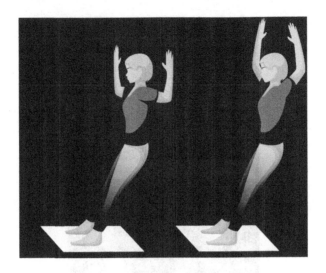

Standing Wall Shoulder Presses

- Keep your back against the wall.
- Your feet should be out a few inches, with your knees slightly bent.
- Keep your arms raised from the elbows up against the wall.
- Elbows should be bent at 90 degrees.
- Remember to keep your movements controlled and focused.
- Do not force or strain.
- Relax and inhale through your nose.
- Exhale through your mouth.
- Slowly raise your arms above your head and keep elbows on the wall if possible.
- Shoulder relaxed and not raised.
- If not, slightly away from the wall.
- Slowly bring your arms back to shoulder-length, raised from the elbows.
- Repeat this five times.

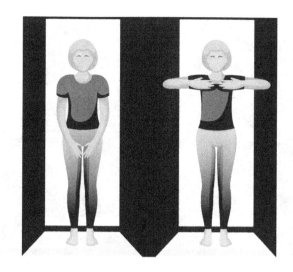

Standing Wall High Pulls

- Stand up straight.
- Keep your back against the wall.
- Abs should be tight, and arms should be straight down, but keep your thumbs and forefingers touching slightly.
- Your feet should be out a few inches and your knees slightly bent.
- Relax and inhale through your nose.
- Exhale through your mouth.
- Lift arms toward shoulders, bending elbows wide, keep hands in front of the body and very close, raise until shoulder height.
- Hold for five counts, then return the hands down.
- Repeat this five times.

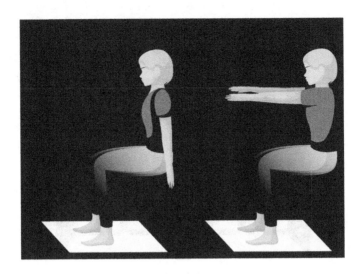

Front Raises in 1/4 Squat

- Keep your back firmly against the wall.
- Your feet should be about 12 inches away from the wall.
- Stand with your arms tight.
- Keep your abs tight.
- Slowly lower your body down the wall as if sitting in a chair and pushing your back against the wall with strong tension.
- Relax and inhale through your nose.
- Exhale through your mouth.
- Be careful not to be on a slippery surface.
- Only go as low as you can.
- It would help if you did not experience any pain or discomfort in your knees.
- Raise both arms straight in front of you, keeping them at shoulder-length.
- Hold for five to ten counts.
- Then raise them wide to the wall, and slowly return down toward the side.
- Then gently raise your body again straight up.
- Take a few deep breaths before repeating this strength exercise five times.

Exercises to Cover for Weeks 2 and 4

Do the following arm stretches during weeks 2 and 4. Do three sets of five to ten repetitions.

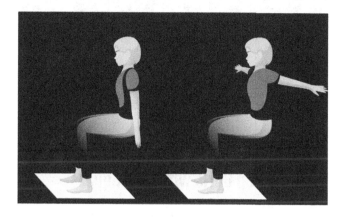

Side Raises with Wall Squats

- This is a partial squat with your back against the wall.
- Keep your back firmly against the wall.
- Your feet should be about 12 inches away from the wall.
- Stand with your arms tight.
- Keep your abs tight.
- Slowly lower your body down the wall as if sitting in a chair and pushing your back against the wall with strong tension.
- Relax and inhale through your nose.
- Exhale through your mouth.
- Be careful not to be on a slippery surface.
- Only go as low as you can.
- It would be best to experience no pain or discomfort in your knees.
- Raise both arms straight horizontally to the side, keeping them at shoulder-length.
- Hold for five to ten counts.
- Then slowly return down toward the side.
- Then gently raise your body again straight up.
- Take a few deep breaths before repeating this strength exercise five times.

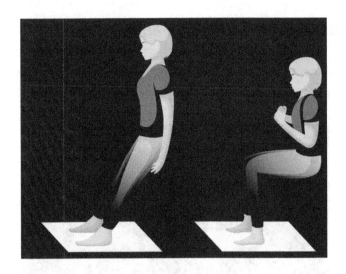

Bicep Curls with Wall Squats

- This is a partial squat with your back against the wall.
- Keep your back firmly against the wall.
- Your feet should be about 12 inches away from the wall.
- Stand with your arms tight on either side, straight down.
- Keep your abs tight.
- Slowly lower your body down the wall as if sitting in a chair and pushing your back against the wall with strong tension.
- Relax and inhale through your nose.
- Exhale through your mouth.
- Be careful not to be on a slippery surface.
- Only go as low as you can.
- It would help if you did not experience any knee pain or discomfort.
- Arms stay down, anchor the elbows, and raise hands up and down.
- Keep your hands in a tight fist as you sit in a squat position.
- Hold for five to ten counts.
- Then slowly return down toward the side.
- Then gently raise your body again straight up.
- Take a few deep breaths before repeating this strength exercise five times.

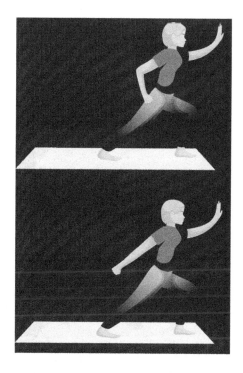

Tricep Kickback in a Split Stance

- Stand facing the wall in a split stance.
- You will place one leg in front of the other.
- The front leg is bent at the knee and the back leg is straight at a 45-degree angle.
- Place one hand on the wall, palm against the wall.
- Keep the extended arm bent at the elbow.
- Relax and inhale through your nose.
- Exhale through your mouth.
- When you're ready, raise the palm of the back arm facing up while raising the arm as high as you can go.
- Do not shrug your shoulders.
- Hold for five to ten counts, then lower the arm back to the start position.
- Repeat this ten times on both sides (on the right side and then on the left side).

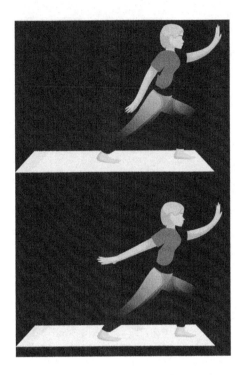

Tricep Lifts in a Split Stance

- Stand facing the wall in a split stance.
- You will place one leg in front of the other.
- The front leg is bent at the knee, and the back leg is straight at a 45-degree angle.
- Place one hand on the wall, palm against the wall.
- Keep the extended arm straight at your side, parallel to the back leg.
- Relax and inhale through your nose.
- Exhale through your mouth.
- When you're ready, raise the back arm with your palm facing down as high as you can go.
- Do not shrug your shoulders.
- Hold for five to ten counts, then lower the arm.
- Repeat this ten times on both sides (to the right side and then to the left side).

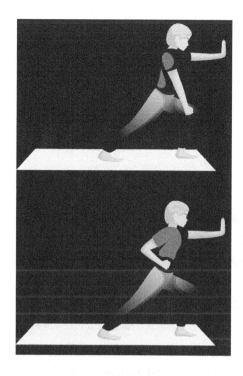

Row in a Split Stance

- Stand facing the wall in a split stance.
- You will place one leg in front of the other.
- The front leg is bent at the knee, and the back leg is straight at a 45-degree angle.
- Place one hand on the wall, palm against the wall.
- Keep the extended arm at your side straight, facing down.
- Relax and inhale through your nose.
- Exhale through your mouth.
- When you're ready, raise the back arm close to your ribcage as if you're squeezing your elbow into your back.
- Do not shrug your shoulders.
- Hold for five to ten counts, then lower the arm straight down.
- Repeat for ten on both sides (to the right and then to the left).

Part E

In this part, we focus on seated arm exercises. These are beneficial for so many reasons, so it's important to highlight them. You will enjoy joint health and there will be a noticeable improvement in balance and stability. When you strengthen your arms this way, you will also benefit from improved posture and reduced risk of falls. If you are suffering from pain due to arthritis, it will help reduce that pain. Finally, these exercises improve muscle rotation and flexibility (Nunez, 2019).

Exercises to Cover for Weeks 1 and 3

Do three sets of the following seated arm exercises with five to ten reps all the way through.

Wall Seated Arm Raises

- Sit flat on your mat with your back against the wall, legs stretched straight out in front of you.
- Bend your knees slightly if necessary.
- Keep your hands straight down to your sides but at a slant with your hands in line with your knees.
- Relax and inhale through your nose.
- Exhale through your mouth.
- When you're ready, raise both arms straight in front of you.
- Hold for three to five counts.
- Then lower them down.
- Repeat ten times.
- Complete three sets.

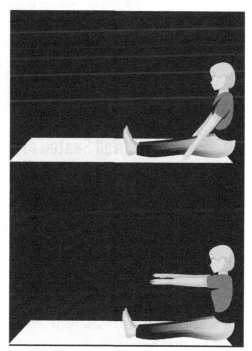

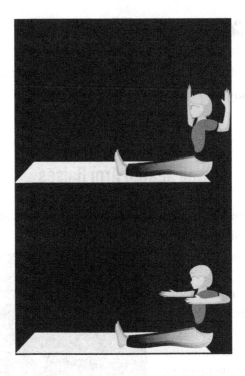

Wall Seated Arm Rotation

- Sit flat on your mat with your back against the wall, legs stretched straight out in front of you.
- Keep your elbows raised to shoulder height.
- Elbows should rest against the wall, shoulder height.
- Forearms stretched in front of you.
- Relax and inhale through your nose.
- Exhale through your mouth.
- When you're ready, raise both arms straight up so that they rest against the wall behind you.
- Hold for three to five counts.
- Then lower them down.
- Repeat ten times.
- Complete three sets.

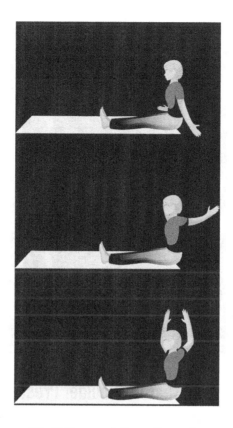

Wall Seated Arm Angels

- Sit flat on your mat with your back against the wall, legs stretched straight out in front of you.
- Keep your palms open and positioned straight to the sides.
- Relax and inhale through your nose.
- Exhale through your mouth.
- When you're ready, raise both arms out wide pressing against the wall (shoulder height) as if you have the wings of an angel.
- Move through the motion smoothly.
- Then raise your arms further up over your head, fully opening up your wings.
- Hold again for three to five counts.
- Then lower them down.
- Repeat ten times.
- Complete three sets.

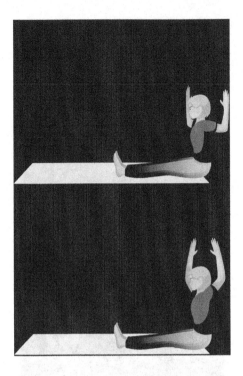

Wall Seated Shoulder Press

- Sit flat on your mat with your back against the wall, legs stretched straight out in front of you.
- Place arms at a 90-degree angle at shoulder height, hands above the bent elbow.
- Relax and inhale through your nose.
- Exhale through your mouth.
- Extend arms overhead keeping elbows against the wall if possible, if not slightly in front of the wall.
- Hold for three to five counts.
- Then lower them down.
- Repeat five to ten times.
- Complete three sets.

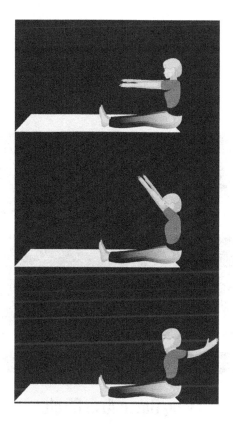

Wall Arm Circles

- Sit flat on your mat with your back against the wall, legs stretched straight out in front of you.
- Keep your hands raised in front of you at shoulder height.
- Relax and inhale through your nose.
- Exhale through your mouth.
- When you're ready, raise both arms as if you are moving them in a circle up to a 45-degree height.
- Move slowly through the motion. Arms don't go behind but circle through the motion.
- Then lower them down, repeating the movements backwards.
- Repeat ten times.
- Complete three sets.

Exercises to Cover for Weeks 2 and 4

Do the following lying-down arm exercises. Do three sets of five to ten reps.

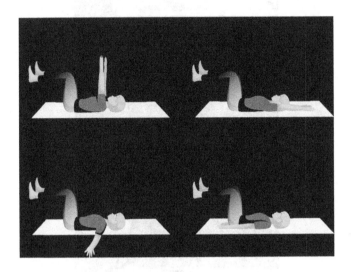

Lying Down Arm Circles

- Lie down on your back with legs raised in a tabletop pose.
- Your knees should be at a 90-degree angle.
- Keep your feet against the wall and relax.
- Inhale through your nose.
- Exhale through your mouth.
- Raise both arms straight up vertically.
- Hold for three to five counts.
- Then move them to the back, placing them flat on the ground behind you.
- Hold again here for five to ten counts.
- Then move your hands horizontally on the ground so that they are aligned straight with your shoulders in a star position.
- Finally, straighten your hands so that they are placed on your sides next to your body, ready to be raised straight up to complete the circle again.
- Repeat ten times.
- Complete three sets.

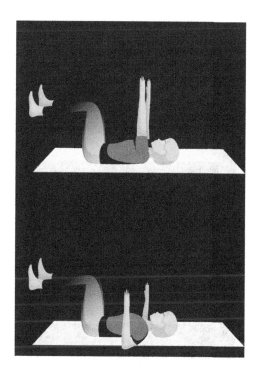

Chest Press

- Lie down on your back with legs raised in a tabletop pose.
- Your knees should be at a 90-degree angle.
- Keep your feet against the wall and relax.
- Inhale through your nose.
- Exhale through your mouth.
- Raise both arms straight up vertically.
- Hold for five to ten counts.
- Then lower them so that they rest on your elbows.
- Repeat ten times.
- Complete three sets.

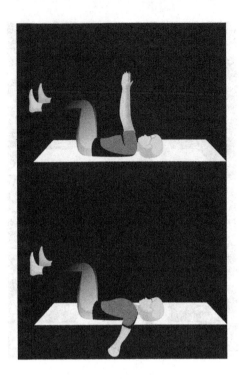

Chest Flies

- Lie down on your back with your legs raised in a tabletop pose.
- Your knees should be at a 90-degree angle.
- Keep your feet against the wall and relax.
- Inhale through your nose.
- Exhale through your mouth.
- Raise both arms straight up vertically.
- Hold for five to ten counts.
- Then lower them completely so that they rest on either side, if possible, and are not strained.
- Repeat ten times.
- Complete three sets.

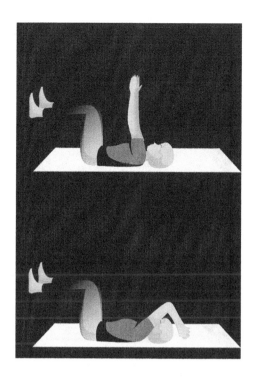

Overhead Tricep Extensions

- Lie down on your back with legs raised in a tabletop pose.
- Your knees should be at a 90-degree angle.
- Keep your feet against the wall and relax.
- Inhale through your nose.
- Exhale through your mouth.
- Raise both arms straight up vertically.
- Hold for three to five counts.
- Then lower them by clasping both hands together and moving down over your head.
- Elbows should be close to your forehead.
- Repeat ten times.
- Complete three sets.

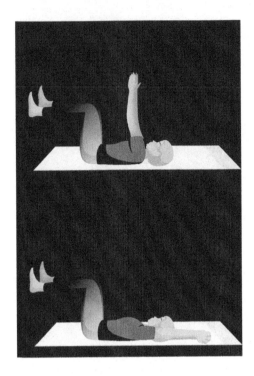

Overhead Reach

- Lie down on your back with legs raised in a tabletop pose.
- Your knees should be at a 90-degree angle.
- Keep your feet against the wall and relax.
- Inhale through your nose.
- Exhale through your mouth.
- Raise both arms straight up vertically.
- Hold for three to five counts.
- Then lower them so that they rest flat on the ground completely behind you.
- Repeat ten times.
- Complete three sets.

Part F

For seniors, maintaining a strong core is important because as we age we lose muscle mass and strength. Strengthening the core helps with posture, prevents injuries, and supports everyday activities. Core muscles support your lower back and also help you to maintain balance. This is vital to ensure strong, confident movements for everyday living (Venkat, 2022).

Exercises to Cover for Weeks 1 to 3

Do the following core exercises for weeks 1 and 3. Make sure you do three sets of five to ten.

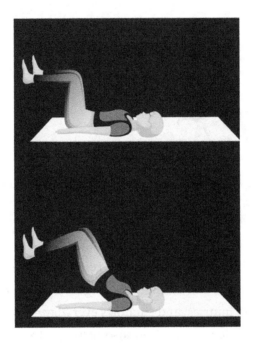

Hip Bridges

- Lie down facing up.
- Bend your legs at your knees with your feet firmly planted on the wall.
- Your feet should be kept hip-width apart.
- Knees bent at a 90-degree angle.
- Raise your hips in the air.
- Contract your glutes as you do this.
- Your arms should be straight and flat on the floor.
- Keep it controlled and focused.
- Relax and inhale through your nose.
- Exhale through your mouth.
- Hold for five to ten counts.
- Repeat five times.

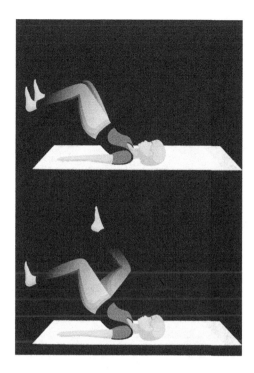

Hip Bridges with Marches

- Lie down facing up.
- Bend your legs at your knees with your feet firmly planted on the wall.
- Your feet should be kept hip-width apart.
- Knees bent at a 90-degree angle.
- Raise your hips in the air.
- Contract your glutes as you do this.
- Your arms should be straight and flat on the floor.
- Then lift one leg to your chest and keep the hips up if possible.
- Alternate the legs and keep the movement controlled.
- Also, keep the spine neutral and the core engaged.
- Relax and inhale through your nose.
- Exhale through your mouth.
- Repeat five times on each leg.

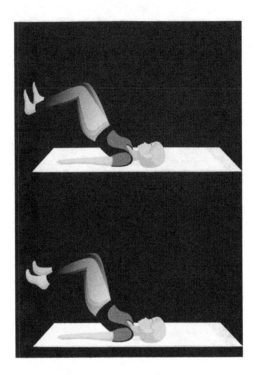

Hip Bridges with Heel Lifts

- Lie down facing up.
- Bend your legs at your knees with your feet firmly planted on the wall.
- Your feet should be kept hip-width apart.
- Knees bent at a 90-degree angle.
- When you're ready, raise your hips in the air.
- Also, raise your heels at the same time.
- Contract your glutes as you do this.
- Your arms should be straight and flat on the floor.
- Keep it controlled and focused.
- Relax and inhale through your nose.
- Exhale through your mouth.
- Lower and lift heels while keeping hips up high, then slowly lower.
- Repeat five times.

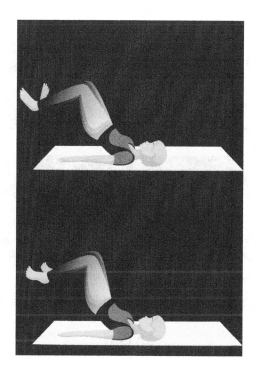

Hip Bridges with Heel Lift Feet in the V Position

- Lie down facing up.
- Bend your legs at your knees with your feet firmly planted on the wall in a V position.
- Your feet should be kept hip-width apart.
- Knees bent at a 90-degree angle.
- Raise your hips in the air as well as your heels.
- Contract your glutes as you do this.
- Your arms should be straight and flat on the floor.
- Keep it controlled and focused.
- Relax and inhale through your nose.
- Exhale through your mouth.
- Lift and lower heels in V then slowly lower.
- Repeat five times.

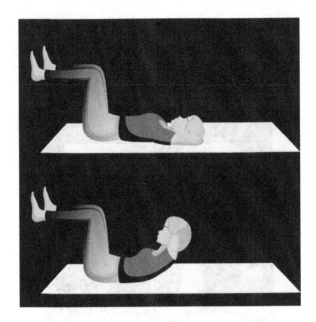

Ab Curl

- Lie down facing up.
- Bend your legs at your knees with your feet firmly planted on the wall.
- Your feet should be kept hip-width apart.
- Knees bent at a 90-degree angle.
- Your hand should be gently supporting your head, not pulling.
- Relax and inhale through your nose.
- Exhale through your mouth.
- When you're ready, raise your head using your abs and not your neck to lift yourself.
- Fix your eyes on the ceiling.
- Keep your chin neutral with your head, about a fist width away from your chest.
- Do ten repetitions of three sets.

Exercises to Cover for Weeks 2 and 4

Do three sets of these core exercises for 10 reps.

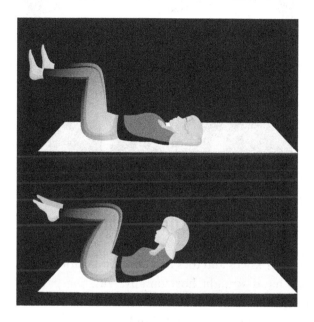

Ab Curl with Knee Tuck

- Lie down facing up.
- Bend your legs at your knees with your feet firmly planted on the wall.
- Your feet should be kept hip-width apart.
- Knees bent at a 90-degree angle.
- Hands should be gently supporting your neck without pulling or straining.
- Relax and inhale through your nose.
- Exhale through your mouth.
- When you're ready, tuck your knees towards your chest as you raise your head simultaneously for an ab curl.
- Remember to keep your core tight by using your abs and not your neck to lift yourself.
- Fix your eyes on the ceiling, keeping your chin up.
- Do ten repetitions of three sets.

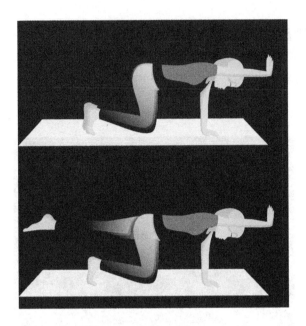

Wall Bird Dog Pointer

- Get onto your knees and toes in a tabletop position.
- Place one hand straight horizontally with the palm of your hand against the wall.
- Raise the opposite leg straight behind you.
- Hold for five to ten counts.
- Relax and inhale through your nose.
- Exhale through your mouth.
- Do ten repetitions on each side for three sets.

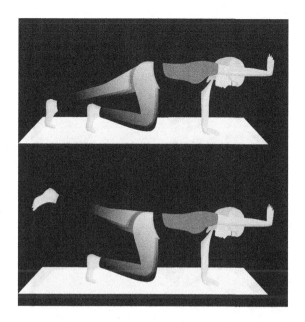

Wall Bird Dog Pointer with Leg Lifts

- Get onto your knees and toes in a tabletop position.
- Place one hand straight horizontally with the palm of your hand against the wall.
- Raise the opposite leg straight behind you.
- Then bring it down and repeat ten times.
- Relax and inhale through your nose.
- Exhale through your mouth.
- Do ten repetitions on each side for three sets.

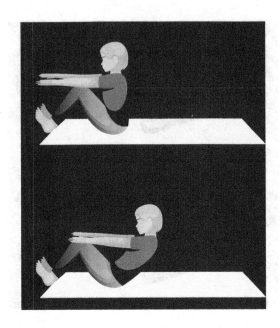

Wall Half Rollbacks

- Sit with your back one foot away from the wall.
- Your knees should be up and your feet against the wall.
- Keep your hands straight in front of you.
- Relax and inhale through your nose.
- Exhale through your mouth.
- Roll back away from the wall and halfway back.
- Then repeat the movement ten times.
- Do three sets.

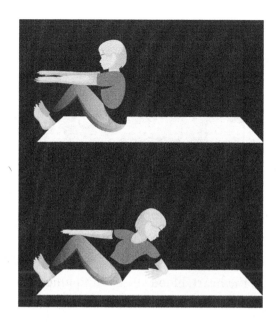

Wall Half Rollbacks with a Twist

- Sit with your back one foot away from the wall.
- Your knees should be up, and your feet should be against the wall.
- Keep your hands straight in front of you.
- Relax and inhale through your nose.
- Exhale through your mouth.
- Roll back away from the wall and twist to one side, hold for five counts.
- Then repeat the movement ten times on both sides.
- Do three sets.

Part G

Cardiovascular exercise is an important component of following a healthy lifestyle. Another word for cardio exercise is "aerobic exercise." It includes many types of exercises that get your heart rate up. This is how you can enhance the efficiency of your cardiovascular system, which comprises the heart, blood vessels, and lungs. They all work together to supply oxygen to your muscles and vital organs. The benefits of engaging in cardio workouts do extend beyond physical fitness. It also positively impacts mental health, significantly contributing to your overall well-being.

The best way to start incorporating cardio into your lifestyle is to find exercises you enjoy. If you're a beginner to cardio workouts, then you need to begin at a comfortable pace. Start at a low impact and take it easy as long as you are comfortable and it is still easy for you to talk or sing as you work out. Let that be the litmus test of what it means to begin doing cardio workouts comfortably. If you have any existing health conditions, it is best that you discuss them with your medical doctor first or with a healthcare professional. Seniors should get at least 30 minutes of cardio exercise (low impact) five days a week. Avoid high-impact cardio exercises. Here are some of the benefits you will enjoy of aerobics exercise (GCS, et al. 2023):

- **Heart health:** Cardio exercise boosts heart health by strengthening the heart muscle. This is what promotes more efficient pumping of blood, which in turn reduces the risk of heart illnesses and diseases.

- **Weight control:** Regular aerobic exercise will help control your weight. Cardio exercises boost weight loss and weight management. It is especially important also to include following a nutritious diet.
- **Improves respiration:** Aerobic exercises are also great for the lungs, improving their capacity to function efficiently.
- **Mood improvement:** Aerobic exercises release dopamine and endorphins in the brain, which are great mood boosters. This, in turn, reduces the production of stress hormones.
- **Better circulation:** aerobic exercises also improve the blood and oxygen flow in the body, thus reducing your chances of developing blood clots.
- **Improved metabolism:** Regular cardio workouts will also boost your metabolism, which is important to burn calories more effectively.
- **Bone health:** You will enjoy improved bone health, which will reduce the likelihood of you suffering from osteoporosis.
- **Joint health:** Regular aerobic exercises also improve joint health. This means that you lower the risk of injuries.
- **Disease prevention:** You can also lower the risk of chronic diseases if you do some type of regular cardio exercise.

Getting started with cardio exercises can be great fun, especially outside. The big gain is, of course, getting some fresh air every day. The exposure also improves mental health. Being outside boosts confidence and also reduces boredom. You can start your cardio journey by doing some easy walking. If you're up to including light jogging in your cardio routine, go for it as long as it feels comfortable. Avoid overexerting yourself. Enjoy some rest periods.

Listen to your body and remember to enjoy the exercises at a comfortable and controlled pace. Here are some aerobic exercises: walking, light jogging, running, swimming, cycling, rope jumping, and water aerobics. Also, do remember to prepare for all weather types. On days when the weather does not permit you to be outside, you can still get a good, solid workout indoors. Here are some indoor aerobic exercises for you to engage in:

- **Marching on the spot:** This is a great way to warm up. You can do this at home or in the garden to get warmed up before indoor cycling, rebounding, or any other low-impact cardio workout. All you need to do is to march in the spot by raising your knees to your chest or as high as you can manage. Alternate the movement of your legs as if you are walking but doing it marching on the spot (*50 Cardio Exercises for Seniors*, 2018).
- **Sidestepping:** This is a wonderful way of firming up the core, legs, and glutes. Do this as part of your warm-up after marching on the spot. You will begin by squatting with your legs wide apart. Don't go too deep with the squat, but enough to be effective. Keep your abs tight, and remember to use your legs and not your hips. Next, you will move your right leg to meet your left leg, then move your left leg to one side and bring your right leg to meet it. Each time, you would take a step to the right and then to the left. You can increase the side-stepping speed or deepen the squat (*50 Cardio Exercises for Seniors*, 2018).
- **Knee raises:** Standing knee raises are a great way of getting your thighs, glutes, and legs in shape. It's also easy to do. You just need to stand with both hands on your hips and raise your knee so your thigh is parallel to the ground. This exercise strengthens your core (*How to Do Standing Knee Raise Exercise with Proper Technique*, n.d.).
- **Step-ups:** You will need an adjustable cardio step for this. Alternatively, you could use a step from your staircase, preferably

the last step at the bottom. You will tap each alternate foot on the step. Start at the bottom of the step, then raise one foot on the step, bring it down, then raise the other foot and keep repeating. (*How to Do Standing Knee Raise Exercise with Proper Technique,* n.d.).

- **Indoor cycling:** This is easy and convenient to do at home, and you will enjoy the benefits of getting some regular cardio exercises into your routine. You will enjoy improved lower body strength, a good cardio workout, and mental health improvements. It is also a great way of keeping fit at home, especially if you love cycling but fear doing it outside on busy streets. Seniors should opt for a recumbent indoor bike as it eases joint stress compared to normal indoor cycling bikes (Walsh, 2023).

- **Using a mini rebounder:** This is a great way to get indoor low-impact cardio workouts. Using a mini rebounder indoors is perfect for any age group, and it does not require you to be at a certain level of fitness. They are easy on the muscles and joints and make cardio workouts less strenuous to some degree. Experts say that despite its low-impact nature, it is a very effective way of strengthening the core, the glutes, and the back. It also helps with balance while stimulating the lymphatic system (Fard, 2022).

- **Dancing to your favorite music:** Dancing to your favorite music will also give you great indoor exercise. Put on your favorite music, enjoy the beat, and dance to your heart's content. This is another great way of achieving a low-impact cardio workout. It can be quite uplifting and good fun too.

Here is a comprehensive overview of the 28-day program; we have broken it down for you into four weeks so that you will know what your focus is every day for each week. You can now prepare yourself mentally and physically for the coming days. You should alternate between upper one day and lower the next day. If you can't get on the floor, then just do all the standing exercises. If getting on the floor is an option, then rotate through standing exercises and floor exercises, being sure to alternate between upper one day and lower the next. Using the above exercises, your four weeks for the 28-day challenge look like this.

Part A: Morning Stretches

	Side-to-side neck stretches
	Ear to shoulder
	Standing side bends
	Standing fold
	Forward hip lunge
	Standing 4 stretches
	Side-facing arm circle
	Standing calf stretch
	Standing arm full circle
	Standing roll downs
	Standing corner chest stretch
	Seated straddle stretch

Part B-Week 1 and 3: Lower Body Standing

Day 1	Standing knee lifts
	Standing leg lift
	Standing leg circle
	Standing leg side lift
	Standing inner thigh lift

Part C-Week 1 and 3: Upper Body Standing

Day 2	Standing wall push-ups (wide)
	Standing wall push-ups (narrow)
	Standing wall shoulder presses
	Standing arms high pulls
	Standing walls front raises in 1/4 squat

Part D-Week 1 and 3: Core

Day 3	Hip bridges
	Hip bridges with marches
	Hip bridges with heel lifts
	Hip bridges in V foot position
	Ab Curl

Day 4: Rest and Stretch Day

Part E-Week 1 and 3: Lower Body on the Floor

Day 5	Bridges on the wall
	Bridges with marches
	Bicycle bridges on the wall
	Bridges with leg circles
	Wall frogs

Part F-Week 1 and 3: Upper Body on the Floor

Day 6	Wall seated arm raise
	Wall seated arm rotation
	Wall seated arm angels
	Wall seated shoulder press
	Wall seated arm circles

Day 7: Rest Day

Part A-Week 2 and 4: Morning Stretches

	Side-to-side neck stretches
	Ear to shoulder
	Standing side bends
	Standing fold
	Forward hip lunge
	Standing 4 stretches
	Side-facing arm circle
	Standing calf stretch
	Standing arm full circle
	Standing to roll down
	Standing corner chest stretch
	Seated straddle stretch

Part B-Week 2 and 4: Lower Body Standing

Day 1	Standing leg hip extension
	Standing leg curls
	Standing wall squats
	Standing wall squats with arm reaches
	Standing lunges toward the wall

Part C-Week 2 and 4: Upper Body Standing

Day 2	Standing wall side raises in 1/4 squat
	Standing wall bicep curls in 1/4 squat
	Tricep kick-back in a split stance
	Tricep Lifts
	One arm row in a split stance

Part D-Week 2 and 4 : Core

Day 3	Ab curl with knee tuck
	Wall bird dog
	Wall bird dog with leg lifts
	Ab half roll back
	Ab half roll back with a twist

Day 4: Rest and Stretch Day

Part E-Week 2 and 4: Lower Body on the Floor

Day 5	Wall splits
	Wall Peter Pan
	Side-lying leg lifts
	Side-lying leg circles
	Side-lying clams

Part F-Week 2 and 4 : Upper Body on the Floor

Day 6	Lying down arm circles
	Lying down chest presses
	Lying down chest fly
	Lying down overhead tricep extensions
	Lying down overhead reach

Day 7: Rest Day

A Suggested Format for the 28-Day Challenge

Here's a recommended structure for the 28-day challenge, but the main goal is to complete it successfully. Remember, there's no competition to finish all exercises in a day if you're feeling fatigued or strained. It's perfectly fine to skip a day, as long as you aim to complete 28 days of exercise within a reasonable timeframe. If you miss a day, that's okay; just ensure you make up for it later. You can always return to the beginning once you've completed the initial round to kick off another 28-day challenge. Keep the momentum going and focus on a long-term commitment to integrating wall Pilates as a significant part of your self-care routine. Also, remember that if you cannot manage to do the floor exercises, stick to the standing ones. I encourage you to include cardio anytime into your routine of your own free will after your wall Pilates daily session. Keep smiling and keep going!

Week 1

Day 1	Lower body standing
Day 2	Upper body standing
Day 3	Core
Day 4	Rest
Day 5	Lower body on the floor
Day 6	Upper body on the floor
Day 7	Rest day

Week 2

Day 1	Lower body standing
Day 2	Upper body standing
Day 3	Core
Day 4	Rest
Day 5	Lower body on the floor
Day 6	Upper body on the floor
Day 7	Rest day

Week 3

Day 1	Lower body standing
Day 2	Upper body standing
Day 3	Core
Day 4	Rest
Day 5	Lower body on the floor
Day 6	Upper body on the floor
Day 7	Rest day

Week 4

Day 1	Lower body standing
Day 2	Upper body standing
Day 3	Core
Day 4	Rest
Day 5	Lower body on the floor
Day 6	Upper body on the floor
Day 7	Rest day

A Quick Recap of Main Points in This Chapter

- A consistent practice of wall Pilates will result in strength, balance, and confidence.
- Pilates is an effective solution for seniors dealing with balance issues.
- It's an effective way to begin your day, as you will be more energized and motivated throughout the day to maintain a healthy, holistic lifestyle.
- Every day for the next four weeks you will stretch, balance, and strengthen core muscles, legs, and arms.
- You now have a weekly exercise schedule to begin the exciting journey of wall Pilates.

You are encouraged to explore these exercises at your own pace. Remember always that it is important to listen to your body and enjoy the process of building strength and flexibility.

WHOLESOME BITES

*R*honda, a dynamic 62-year-old business owner, navigated long and sometimes stressful days, leaving her tired and mentally drained. She sighed as she contemplated her busy schedule and realized that years had flown by. When she got home, she hurriedly ate dinner and went to bed exhausted from the day's events. This realization sparked a desire for change within her. During her college days, Rhonda was once athletic and studious, but she also made time to hang out with friends in beautiful natural settings. She missed those carefree days of having fun and relaxing while listening to the sounds of a flowing river.

As she reflected on her past and compared it to her current lifestyle, Rhonda felt the need to reclaim her vitality. However, she faced the challenge of not knowing where to begin. A close friend suggested that she prioritize her health and wellness as a starting point for adjusting. With no regular physical exercise, she decided it would be a great place to start. In addition to starting a new exercise routine, Rhonda embarked on a journey to reclaim her health by significantly changing her diet. She delved deep into balanced nutrition as someone who pays attention to detail. She found herself immersed in various books, seeking knowledge about the impact of different foods on her energy levels.

It was crucial for Rhonda to feel more energized and radiate good health from within. She envisioned her skin glowing and her vital organs thriving. This was how she expressed her goal to her friends. Her first step towards achieving this was eliminating processed foods from her diet. She also aimed to reduce her consumption of red meat. Rhonda recognized that she needed to consider the potential risks associated with adults over 65 to reclaim her vitality. Her commitment to making these changes grew stronger when she learned about how the food choices of seniors could impact their heart health, bone strength, and brain function (Ortiz, 2018).

Rhonda was aware of the potential risks of consuming excessive red meat, especially for those over 65. Studies have shown that it can contribute to the development of colon cancer and raise the risk of Alzheimer's disease (Ortiz, 2018). She wanted to avoid associating her golden years with the fear of poor health. Rhonda aimed to find a balance between enjoying life, caring for her health, and maintaining her happiness and wisdom. She recognized that being overweight was not an option either, as it can lead to conditions such as diabetes, strokes, and weak bone health. Rhonda started replacing processed foods with nourishing whole foods to gradually transition to a healthier lifestyle.

She increased her intake of fruits, vegetables, and lean proteins while also incorporating whole grains into her diet. After just a few weeks, she noticed a remarkable transformation. She felt more energized, and her mental well-being improved. It became evident to her that what we eat significantly impacts how we feel. Rhonda understood the importance of listening to her body's signals, just as she would during exercise.

She recognized that a healthy diet benefits physical health and plays a crucial role in managing stress, improving concentration, enhancing self-esteem, and promoting better mental health (Mental Health Including Anxiety and Depression, 2020).

As the weeks went by, Rhonda underwent a remarkable transformation. She felt a significant increase in her energy levels and improved overall mood. This newfound energy allowed her to exercise more and spend quality time with her family. Dinners were no longer rushed, and the table became adorned with vibrant and healthy salads as important side dishes. Rhonda incorporated fruit into her snacks throughout the day and allowed herself occasional indulgences while maintaining a focus on moderation. She became mindful of the quality of food she consumed, attributing all the positive changes to her health and vitality to this profound shift in her dietary choices.

Rhonda's story underscores the important lesson that proper nutrition complements physical exercise. She experienced the importance of fueling her body with the right food combinations to boost her energy levels. The transformative power of following a balanced nutritional eating plan for seniors became evident to her. By making intentional choices about the foods she ate, she discovered that she could enhance her energy levels and support her rest and recovery phase. This renewed sense of vitality brought new light and vibrancy to her life. Following a healthy diet became the guiding light that led her into the best years of her life. Let's now explore the core principles of nutrition for seniors and uncover carefully considered strategies that will serve you well!

Fundamentals of Nutrition

As we journey through aging, our needs evolve. For example, Rhonda has grown tired of the endless busy hours at work. It was taking a toll on her health. The signs of exhaustion were apparent. It became clear that as we age, we must cultivate a lifestyle that restores lost vitality and prioritizes nourishing our minds and bodies. When we feel good from the inside out, our spirits soar. Just as you've been encouraged to follow a more holistic approach to exercise, the same principle applies to your dietary requirements. Consider the food you consume as an opportunity to fuel positivity within you. Processed foods, on the other hand, do not provide this nourishment. They can leave you feeling sluggish and impact your mood, ultimately leading to a decline in physical health. As seniors, it is vital to adopt a diet that directly addresses our specific health concerns, including bone health, organ functioning, and immunity.

As we recognize the decline in brain health associated with aging, it becomes crucial to prioritize foods that support cognitive function. Shifting to a healthier lifestyle is not a complicated task. It begins with understanding your body's nutritional requirements and selecting natural foods rich in these essential nutrients. Powering up naturally means shifting away from processed foods and incorporating a mix of fruits, vegetables, lean proteins, whole grains, and healthy fats. These nutrient-dense foods support vital processes such as digestion, immunity, and cognitive function. Adopting a balanced and nutritious approach can reduce the risk of feeling exhausted or mentally drained and sustain your energy throughout the day. It is also important to recognize how embracing a health-conscious lifestyle, particularly focusing on your body's nutritional needs, can enhance your exercise sessions, such as the wall Pilates journey.

Eating clean and nourishing foods will energize you and deepen your holistic approach to well-being. By acknowledging the synergistic relationship between nutrition and exercise, you will experience an amazing sense of well-being from the inside out. Feeling good is an inside-out journey that requires taking stock of your lifestyle and making significant changes to allow for transformation. A well-balanced diet boosts energy levels and enhances the enjoyment you derive from your daily exercise routine, revitalizing your overall health. When you prioritize your body's nutritional needs, you also reap the rewards of an improved immune system, enhanced cognitive health, and a reduced risk of chronic diseases. Let's now delve deeper into the specific nutritional requirements for seniors and explore the key principles that will guide us toward optimum health (*Nutrition for Older Adults*, n.d.).

Key points: How to Eat Healthy as Your Age

Let's look at the key points of our discussion so far. To eat healthy, you can make the following adjustments immediately. These adjustments are not hard to make. It's only a question of shifting your priority and making new choices when you shop (*Nutrition for Older Adults*, n.d.):

- **Eat foods loaded with nutritional value, such as:**
  - fruits and vegetables
  - whole grains like brown rice, oats, quinoa
  - fat-free dairy products
  - vegetarian dairy
  - fat-free cheeses
  - seafood
  - lean meats
  - poultry and eggs
  - nuts and seeds
  - legumes
- **Avoid empty calories, mostly found in processed foods:** Stay away from them as far as possible. They are chips, sodas, baked sugary desserts, alcohol, all-fried foods, and processed meats.
- **Choose foods that contain lower fat and cholesterol levels:** You should completely avoid trans fat and saturated fats. Pizzas,

and fried foods, like fried chicken, doughnuts, pastries, pies, pie crust, and cookie dough to name but a few, contain trans fats. Also, avoid margarine and vegetable shortening. These contain saturated fats.

- **Drink water:** Make sure that you stay hydrated throughout the day. At the very least, you should aim to drink at least eight glasses of water a day. As we age, our bodies require more water to regulate our body's temperature. It is important to be aware of the risk of dehydration. Water can also fight off other health issues. When you work out, make sure that you are sipping water in between your exercises (hicks, 2020).
- **Exercise regularly:** It cannot be stressed enough how important it is for you to get regular exercise. Exercise improves your immune system; prevents disease, and improves mental health, and cognition (*Five Benefits of Exercise for Seniors*, 2016).

Key Nutrients for Seniors

You can use the following as a guide to ensure that you are getting all of these nutrients in your body daily. Remember that everyone is unique, so we may have unique nutritional requirements. It is important to consult with a medical expert. Here are the basic guidelines (Dodd, 2020):

- **Calcium and vitamin D:** They are both essential for bone health. As we age, they become even more important. Taking a regular dose of both can help maintain strong bone density and reduce the risk of fractures and osteoporosis.
- **Protein:** This is essential for maintaining muscle mass, so make sure to consume enough lean protein daily. It not only helps you feel strong and capable but also aids in post-workout recovery. Protein shakes are a good source of lean protein and fiber. For

seniors, it is advisable to include lean meats, eggs, and poultry in their daily diet in reasonable portions to meet their protein needs and promote overall well-being.

- **Fiber:** plays a crucial role in improving digestion and promoting gut health. It aids in preventing constipation. Fiber also keeps you regular. You can increase your fiber intake by prioritizing consuming more fresh fruits and vegetables and whole-grain foods. These nutritious choices provide essential vitamins and minerals and contribute to a healthy digestive system.

- **Omega-3 fatty acids:** These are beneficial for heart health and have anti-inflammatory properties. Including sources of omega-3 fatty acids in your diet can have positive effects on your overall well-being. Opt for foods such as fatty fish like salmon, trout, and sardines. Also, add walnuts and flaxseeds. These are excellent sources of these essential fatty acids. Omega-3 fatty acids help to support cardiovascular health.

- **B vitamins:** These essential nutrients play a crucial role in brain health. B Vitamins are vital for maintaining cognitive function and a healthy nervous system. You can find B vitamins in a variety of foods. They include whole grains, lean proteins, such as poultry and fish, as well as leafy green vegetables like spinach and broccoli.

- **Boosting your nutritional intake with supplements:** This can be a convenient way to ensure you are getting all the necessary nutrients. Supplements can provide your daily dose of nutrition and fill any potential gaps in your diet. However, it is important to consult with your healthcare provider before starting any new supplements, as they can provide personalized recommendations based on your specific needs and health conditions.

- **Cut down on salt (sodium)**

Below is a table to further help you distinguish between the best and worst food choices you can make for yourself. Look out for the "healthy foods to avoid."

Best foods	Worst foods	Healthy foods to avoid
Fresh colorful vegetables	Foods that contain high sugar content	Processed juices with high sugar content
Fresh fruit	Beverages that can have a high sugar content	High caffeinated drinks
Berries	Processed foods high in sodium, like canned foods and processed meats	Raw seafood (or undercooked)
Nuts and seeds	Food that contains high levels of saturated and trans fats	Yogurts with a high sugar content
Fatty fish and whole grains	Excessive red meat (choose small portions with no fat)	Food high in sodium

When modifying your diet, remember that it can be a gradual journey. It's perfectly acceptable to begin with minor adjustments. It is recommended to adhere to the aforementioned approach as closely as possible. Acknowledge the small triumphs and concentrate on integrating subtle alterations into your daily routine. For instance, if you fondly love cake, consider reducing your intake rather than eliminating it. Avoid consuming cake daily; instead, indulge in moderation on occasion, and explore sugar-free or healthier alternatives made with almond flour, coconut flour, and fresh fruit. Your dedication will be handsomely rewarded, and you'll experience a remarkable boost in energy levels, leaving you feeling fantastic.

A Quick Recap of Main Points in This Chapter

- Mental and physical wellness is largely determined by your choice of foods.
- Consuming food that is full of essential nutrients will increase your energy level while reducing the risk of disease.
- Seniors need to ensure that they are getting their daily intake of nutritional requirements to improve cognitive functions.
- Staying hydrated with water throughout the day is essential for seniors, as more water is required to moderate the body's temperature.
- Snack on fruits and vegetables to obtain nutrition for the body.
- Reducing both sodium and sugar intake is an essential way of staying energized and healthy.
- The types of food we consume determine our mood and how we think.
- Positivity is associated with nutrient-rich food and exercise.

Let's reflect on what we've just learned about making healthier food choices and making a daily connection between good nutrition and following an active lifestyle. Another tenet of a healthy lifestyle is sleep—getting a good night's rest will be the focus of Chapter 7.

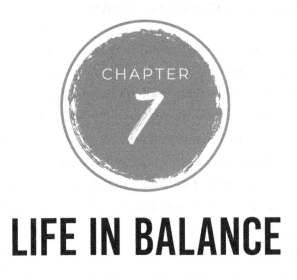

CHAPTER

7

LIFE IN BALANCE

$\mathcal{S}$usan, who recently turned 61, had always been an active and vibrant individual, but recently, she was struggling with sleep disturbances. Initially, she dismissed it. However, as it persisted in her life, she took a moment to reflect on how it affected her physical and mental well-being. She decided to find a solution and began exploring the concept of sleep hygiene. She discovered valuable insights about her current lifestyle and realized the need to adopt healthier habits to ensure uninterrupted sleep. You might be curious about what sleep hygiene entails and how to incorporate it into your routine for a restful sleep. Our bodies and minds deserve deep and peaceful rest after a long day, and our daily choices ultimately influence our sleep patterns.

Sleep hygiene involves being mindful of your daily lifestyle and adopting habits that facilitate quality sleep. It entails cultivating routines and a lifestyle that promotes uninterrupted sleep. Susan recognized that her current lifestyle was not conducive to practicing good sleep hygiene, which hurt her sleep patterns. She made deliberate changes to experience a more restful and peaceful sleep. One of the first adjustments she made was establishing a consistent bedtime. Additionally, Susan decided to avoid consuming coffee at night, as she had developed a dependence on it, which occasionally hindered her ability to achieve deep rest.

Seniors are particularly advised to limit their caffeine intake throughout the day. Especially in the evening, it is recommended to abstain from consuming coffee—for at least three hours before bedtime. Caffeine can potentially prolong wakefulness, making it difficult to fall asleep. This is due to its stimulating effects, promoting alertness rather than sleepiness. Insomnia, the inability to sleep, can occur when caffeine is consumed in excessive quantities. The impact of caffeine on sleep quality depends on the amount and timing of consumption. When consumed in high doses, caffeine blocks the receptors that induce sleep with a chemical called Adenosine, leading to sleep disturbances. This is how caffeine can interfere with a sound night's sleep, leaving you tossing and turning in bed with a racing mind filled with multiple thoughts (Pacheco & Cotliar, 2021).

Establishing Sleep Hygiene

Susan embarked on her sleep hygiene journey by establishing a consistent bedtime routine. In the two hours leading up to sleep, she engaged in reading a captivating book, allowing her mind to unwind. She enjoyed a warm bath and incorporated soothing essential oils like lavender and eucalyptus to enhance relaxation. In the evening, she dimmed the lights and added the ambiance of candles to create a tranquil atmosphere, which helped prevent excessive rumination on the day's events. Susan observed significant improvements in her sleep quality.

Occasionally, she dedicated 20 minutes to unwinding in her hot tub, accompanied by gentle meditation music, relieving stress and letting go of the day's demands and responsibilities. Mornings brought Susan a sense of alertness, refreshment, and enthusiasm to embrace the new day. She felt invigorated and healthier by starting her day with a nutritious breakfast of fruits and a bowl of oats. Rather than immediately reaching for her favorite cup of coffee, she opted for warm water with lemon or a soothing cup of tea.

She also took a few moments to sit outside in her garden, breathing in the fresh air. With her newfound energy, Susan dedicated her vitality to practicing Pilates, specifically wall Pilates, in the mornings. This positive choice had multiple benefits. She joined a local Pilates class and committed herself to regular practice. Little did she know that her dedication to Pilates would further enhance her sleep patterns. The combination of physical exercise, stretching, and relaxation techniques enabled Susan to achieve an even deeper and more rejuvenating sleep.

Wall Pilates Is Best Done in the Mornings

Engaging in wall Pilates in the mornings offers a wide range of benefits. However, it's important to note that exercise can be beneficial at any time of the day. One of the key advantages of practicing wall Pilates in the mornings, particularly for seniors, is that it provides a fantastic way to start the day. It generates energy and motivation, inspiring individuals to maintain healthier daily habits. Morning exercise, including wall Pilates, has enhanced participants' mood, metabolism, and alertness. Establishing a morning exercise routine creates a positive tone for the day.

For seniors, a morning workout can help combat lethargy and lack of motivation. It also promotes joint lubrication, increased blood flow, enhanced flexibility, and reduced pain and stiffness. This makes it particularly advantageous for seniors to engage in a morning exercise routine, reaping the benefits of improved overall well-being. There's nothing quite like a good stretch to alleviate any bodily aches and pains. Whether you ask seniors or individuals of any age, they will attest to the incredible feeling of endorphins and dopamine flooding the bloodstream. These chemicals, found in the brain, play a vital role in regulating mood and emotional well-being.

Dopamine is often referred to as the "feel-good" hormone, while endorphins are known as the "happy hormone." It is essential to have a healthy dose of both for increased productivity, happiness, and positivity. Exercise is a natural way to stimulate these positive feelings and emotions. When you exercise, your body rewards you by producing these wonderful chemicals, creating a natural high. It's hard to argue against starting your day on such a delightful note. Research also shows that people who exercise regularly experience lower stress levels than those who do not.

Chemically, the body responds by producing lower levels of stress hormones known as cortisol and epinephrine. This is fantastic because higher levels result in anxiety, irritability, and intense emotions associated with the fight or flight response to stressful situations or negative thoughts (*Working Out Boosts Brain Health*, 2020). Wall Pilates is an important reason for waking up in the morning motivated to honor your body and health and seize the day with enthusiasm. It enhances feelings of being present and in control. The morning sunlight beaming into your room is yet another compelling reason to embrace a morning session of wall Pilates. Exposure to natural light also has a positive influence on sleep patterns.

That's because exposure to natural sunlight synchronizes our internal body clock. This is known as the Circadian Rhythm Regulation. This refers to the 24-hour cycles that become part of our body's internal clock system. When exposed to the morning light, your circadian rhythm shifts accordingly and becomes synchronized with nature, so you may start to feel sleepy by sunset. In other words, your internal clock becomes synchronized with the external light. When you set your internal biological clock this way by synchronizing it with nature, you are more inclined to experience a deep, restful, and restorative sleeping pattern.

That is why waking up in the morning to feel and experience the first rays of sunshine and have a good workout is a wonderful way of programming your body to rest well in the evenings. Circadian rhythms are also believed to impact mental and physical well-being (Suni, 2023). It's time now to turn our attention to some of the most common sleep challenges faced by seniors. The more awareness we have of this, the greater our chances of overcoming it.

Common Sleep Problems Experienced by Seniors

As you go through the natural process of aging, your lifestyle and habits do change. Our sleeping patterns also change as we age. But now you know that it remains important for your well-being to get a good night's rest. Here are the common sleep problems associated with aging (*Sleep Disorders in Older Adults: MedlinePlus Medical Encyclopedia*, 2017):

- **Insomnia:** Refers to the difficulty that we experience in falling asleep at night. Insomnia usually results in fatigue during the day.
- **Sleep apnea:** This condition is best described as paused breathing that occurs at night during your sleep. It can severely disrupt the quality of your sleep.
- **Restless Legs Syndrome (RLS):** It refers to an uncomfortable sensation in your legs. You will feel the urge to keep moving your legs to fall asleep properly.

- **Periodic Limb Movement Disorder (PLMD):** You may find that your legs keep moving while you're asleep involuntarily. This is quite disturbing and breaks a healthy sleeping pattern.
- **REM Sleep Behavior Disorder (RBD):** This occurs when there is a loss of muscle relaxation during REM sleep. This can result in vivid dreams or even violent dreams in some situations.
- **Circadian Rhythm Disorders:** When disruptions occur in the internal body clock, it may result in difficulties falling asleep.

Managing Stress for a Balanced Life

Throughout life's journey, we encounter a series of challenges that shape us and test our resilience. From the early stages of learning to crawl and walk, to the rebellious teenage years where we explore our identities, and the responsibilities that come with adulthood, we face a multitude of hurdles. However, as seniors, we confront unique challenges associated with aging and the latter part of our lives.

One of the major sources of stress among seniors is the uncertainty of their health. The fear of age-related illnesses looms ever-present, leaving us feeling vulnerable and dependent on others for care. Financial instability is another common stressor, as we must navigate the complexities of finding purposeful employment or relying on others for support. This can lead to feelings of anxiety and emotional strain, diminishing our sense of independence and control.

Social isolation and loneliness can also have a significant impact on our well-being. The loss of meaningful connections and the freedom to live life on our terms can leave us feeling isolated and demotivated. Loneliness may even contribute to making poor health choices and slipping into a state of depression.

To regain a sense of purpose, inspiration, and joy, it is crucial to take control of our lives once more. Managing stress becomes essential in navigating through these challenges. While moments of frustration are inevitable, the key lies in pulling ourselves out of these low points, healing, and adapting to a new lifestyle. It is important to accept that behind every challenge, hidden blessings are waiting to be discovered.

To better handle stress as it arises in our lives, here are some strategies that can be beneficial:

- Prioritize self-care by engaging in activities that bring joy and relaxation.
- Maintain a strong support network of friends and family who can provide emotional support.
- Practice mindfulness and embrace the present moment to cultivate a sense of inner calm.
- Seek professional help or guidance through therapy or counseling if needed.
- Stay physically active and adopt healthy lifestyle habits to boost mental and physical well-being.
- Cultivate a positive mindset by focusing on gratitude and finding the silver linings in challenging situations.

Remember, stress management is an essential component of navigating the unique challenges that seniors face. By proactively addressing stress, we can strive towards a more fulfilling and joyful life in our senior years.

A Quick Recap of Main Points in This Chapter

- Sleep hygiene is important for seniors.
- It involves developing healthier habits to ensure uninterrupted sleep.

- If you are experiencing sleep issues, you should consult with a professional to get to the root cause of the problem. It could be related to your lifestyle.
- Prioritize daily self-care activities, including wall Pilates to bring about relaxation and restful sleep at night.
- Take care of your stress levels because this too impacts health, wellness, and sleeping patterns.
- Ultimately aims at cultivating a positive mindset to achieve greater feelings of personal fulfillment.

Remember that following a balanced lifestyle is key to maximizing the benefits of Pilates and improving the overall quality of life for seniors.

CHAPTER

8

EBB AND FLOW OF MOTIVATION

*S*heryl initially found herself discouraged by her slow progress in wall Pilates. It's natural to feel discouraged, but it's important not to let that get in the way. Recognize that the mind and body are adjusting to change and that initial discomfort is to be expected when stepping out of your comfort zone. It's also beneficial to set realistic expectations for yourself. Sheryl's disappointment stemmed from being too hard on herself. Remember, there is nothing to prove to yourself or anyone else. Instead, embrace wall Pilates as a positive addition to your life and aim to enjoy each session.

Throughout our lives, we have been conditioned to prove ourselves in the world constantly. However, when responsibilities pile up, we become even harder on ourselves. Instead of pushing yourself, ease into a new routine and remember that consistency is key to achieving your health goals. On days when you feel a bit off, it's important to understand that it doesn't mean you haven't made any progress. Take that day off, rest, or immerse yourself in activities you love, such as cooking a delicious meal, baking, gardening, or any activity that brings you tranquility and joy. Remember to prioritize self-care and seek moments of peace amidst the journey towards better health.

Sheryl decided to take up wall Pilates with high hopes, and naturally, she felt disappointed when she realized that she wasn't living up to the high ideals and expectations she had set for herself. Remembering that self-love involves accepting yourself completely, just as you are now, is important. The key is to pour acceptance and love into every cell of your body, which allows you to become more present and grounded. Recognizing that fantasies and unrealistic expectations can lead to unnecessary pressure and the need to prove oneself to others is important. Instead, focus on finding joy in every moment of your life, embracing the natural flow of things.

This mindset applies to any significant changes you make, including your exercise routine. Approach these changes gracefully and with ease, knowing that each day brings a shift in the quality of your life and health. Sheryl's disappointment arose from the misalignment between her expectations and realistic goals. It's crucial to acknowledge that motivation naturally fluctuates, and this is a normal part of the process. Rather than relying on constant high motivation, it is essential to prioritize sticking to your daily exercise routine and embracing the countless benefits it brings. By going with the flow and maintaining consistency, you can be kind to yourself and understand that fluctuations in motivation are inherent to the journey.

In Sheryl's case, she exemplified determination and resilience. She refused to give up easily and actively worked on shifting her mindset and approaching her wall Pilates journey. Sheryl realized that she could achieve her goals by easing into a gentle routine and finding joy in each stretch and movement of her body. During this process, Sheryl became aware of the negative clutter in her mind and recognized the need to address the root cause of her high expectations. By shifting to a positive mindset, she discovered that she had been expecting herself to fail, which led her to push herself excessively and mask it with an outward display of high enthusiasm. Sheryl realized that our minds can sometimes deceive us, and it's important to let go of everything and embrace an inspiring new routine.

The foundation of positivity lies in following an inspiring exercise routine that honors the body, mind, and spirit. Sheryl learned to appreciate herself for embarking on these gentle changes that would rejuvenate and bring vitality back into her life. She embarked on a transformative journey toward holistic well-being by embracing this mindset. Sheryl started setting small, realistic goals instead of being inauthentic to herself. She wanted to learn each pose and master it to ensure alignment, posture, and breath control. Above all else, she wanted to be completely relaxed in the present moment of pure enjoyment. As Sheryl started implementing these changes, there was a notable shift in her attitude.

She started feeling a renewed sense of enjoyment and inner peace. She was also more accepting of herself and began nurturing this renewed sense of calm and positivity. She focused on the journey itself and not a fantasy of how things would be. She wanted to count the blessings of each day and connect with herself deeply to appreciate both the internal and external changes taking place as a result of the new healthy habits that she was forming. Slowly, but surely, she began to see improvements in her abilities. Over time, her persistence and positive mindset set in motion the lasting changes she wanted to experience every day from all the healthy changes she made.

The significant lesson from Sheryl's story is the value of self-awareness in adjusting our mindset to support our goals, especially when our motivation lags behind our progress. It is essential to recognize that our minds may need to readjust to a more realistic outlook, founded on self-acceptance. By embracing the entire journey, we can cultivate a positive mindset that will ultimately transform our exercise experience. Perseverance, achievement, and positivity are interconnected. As you make significant changes to your lifestyle, view these as the three pillars of your ongoing success.

Another important lesson from Sheryl's story is the recognition that practicing supportive and encouraging self-talk is crucial in the face of challenges. Additionally, it is advisable to approach goal setting conservatively. While it's important to maintain a larger vision in mind, breaking it down into small, achievable goals is essential. By doing so, you can stay motivated and track your progress effectively. Setting small, achievable goals helps to build momentum and confidence, making it easier to stay motivated.

By embracing the journey and focusing on the process rather than solely on the result, you can find more enjoyment in your journey. I encourage you to celebrate every milestone of your journey towards reclaiming health and vitality. This will help you stay inspired and motivated to keep moving in the right direction, preserving physical, mental, and emotional wellness. A positive mindset not only enhances physical performance but also builds mental resilience, allowing setbacks to be seen as opportunities for growth. It's important to acknowledge that motivation naturally fluctuates, especially on those days when things don't seem to be going your way. Instead of feeling burdened by setbacks, try to recognize and accept these fluctuations.

Instead of dwelling on negative thoughts, let go of the urge to entertain them and focus on moving forward. Consider journaling to document your thoughts, feelings, progress, setbacks, and successes. For instance, after a week, note any improvements in your mood, decreased stress levels, or reduced worry. By writing down these positive experiences, you can reflect on your progress at any time. Journaling is a valuable outlet for expressing thoughts and feelings, allowing them to be released. It also provides an opportunity to contemplate personal growth, mindset shifts, and physical changes. Take a moment to examine your thoughts and feelings about the journey ahead. Use the space below to start journaling.

Journal Entry: Thoughts and Feelings About the Journey

1.

2.

3.

4.

5.

6.

7.

8.

9.

10.

Take a moment to write down all the reasons why you are embarking on this journey to reclaim vitality. By documenting your motivations, you can reflect on them as you make progress. Keep this journal in a place that is easily accessible and visible, serving as a daily reminder of the commitment you are making to your body, mind, and spirit. Start your journal now and ensure that you use it to track your daily progress, expressing gratitude to your body for the effort it is putting in.

Journal Entry: Thoughts and Feelings About the Journey

1.

2.

3.

4.

5.

6.

7.

8.

9.

10.

Staying the Course

Starting a fitness journey, particularly with wall Pilates, is an excellent first step towards holistic wellness. For seniors facing challenges related to movement, flexibility, joint and muscle pain, and posture issues, wall Pilates offers a wonderful opportunity to regain control and address these concerns daily. As discussed in Chapter 5, I have simplified the approach while ensuring its effectiveness, guiding you toward fitness, flexibility, strength, and balance. It's common to feel highly motivated at the beginning of a new endeavor, but it's important to maintain that motivation throughout. To stay consistent, consider setting daily goals instead of weekly or monthly ones.

Here are some tips to maintain or reignite motivation, coupled with strong mental exercises (McCoy, 2023):

- **Set daily goals:** Commit to taking things one day at a time, one step at a time. See each new day as a brand-new opportunity to be amazing and feel amazing. Even if you experience low-energy days, stretch for at least five minutes and give yourself a pat on the back.
- **Positive self-talk:** It's not difficult for most people to think negative thoughts. So cultivate the practice of thinking positive thoughts. When you catch yourself being negative, strike it out and replace it with positive words. For example, you can change thoughts of giving up to thoughts of trying again tomorrow when your mood is better.
- **Choose a variety of exercises:** Keep your Pilates routine exciting by introducing new movements or hop online and try out one with an online instructor. You can find wall Pilates workouts for seniors on YouTube to spice things up. Throw in a deep guided meditation to boost your levels of positivity when you're feeling down, instead of allowing negativity to take control of your choices and life.
- **Get some outside help:** You can join a mat Pilates class for seniors in your neighborhood or local gym or get a few friends together for your daily classes and take turns on who will be hosting it each day to make it fun and keep the momentum

going. Even if it is a Pilates get-together once a week to work on your movements—that could be fun.

- **Celebrate the milestones:** Instead of only focusing on long-term goals, set achievable milestones. For example, you can opt to reward yourself at least once a week for your efforts, as long as you stick to it four or five times a week. Treat yourself out to lunch, or a day at the spa. When you celebrate milestones, you're reinforcing positive habits and turning your exercising into a source of pleasure and joy.
- **Embrace baby steps:** This means that you should avoid following an all-or-nothing approach to your new routine. Remember that all small steps add up as they gain momentum and lead to longer-term transformation. If you miss a day, you miss a day. Don't stress over it. Count the little blessings and the baby steps that you're taking. Making some regular effort is better than making no effort.

A Quick Recap of Main Points in This Chapter

- Motivation fluctuates, so accept that on some days you will be stronger, while on other days you may not even want to look at the wall.
- Strive to be consistent as long as you have the energy to do so. Make it to the wall and do something, even if it's only half of the session.
- Missing classes because you may not be feeling up to it is okay. Giving up altogether is quitting.
- Allow yourself a period of grace now and then and don't even think about it.

- Chill out with your friends and share the news about your wall Pilates routine. Maybe you can start a wall Pilates group get-together to keep your motivation levels up.

To sustain unwavering motivation despite potential fluctuations, maintain a positive mindset and unwavering consistency. Embrace your journey as a sacred path to honor your body, and remember to document your thoughts, experiences, and triumphs in a journal.

CONCLUSION

The only way to bring about effective and powerful transformation is to dive in and do it. You have a powerful formula in your hands now, and it will transform your life in 28 days. Are you up for the challenge? I hope that you answered strongly in the affirmative. I assure you that following a daily stretching and exercise routine is an effective path for your health. Many seniors hesitate to jump right in at first. Resistance is expected. This is why I wrote this book, to answer your questions by explaining as succinctly as possible all the gains you will encounter from exercising daily. Primarily, the initial hesitation often stems from a lack of sufficient information.

My goal is to bridge that knowledge gap by crafting a comprehensive 28-day program that will set you on the path to improved health and overall wellness. Additionally, I aim to dispel the myths surrounding aging that often hinder seniors from taking full control of their physical well-being. Opting for a sedentary lifestyle is not an option. You have the power to challenge those misconceptions. Common beliefs, such as being too weak for exercise or fearing it will worsen existing pain, can be debunked. It's crucial to consult with a healthcare professional before starting, and your trusted doctor is the best source for personalized advice on the exercises recommended in this book.

These exercises are not just powerful and challenging but also highly effective, designed over four weeks to enhance strength, flexibility, balance, and toning. You owe it to yourself to lead an extraordinary life, even during your golden years, where the celebration of life should continue. Regular exercise can revive lost vitality, uplift mental well-being, and infuse a newfound zest that may have eluded you in the past. Wall Pilates stands out as a cherished holistic approach to exercise for seniors. The radiant vitality, courtesy of endorphins and dopamine, is truly invaluable. Consider wall Pilates as more than just an exercise routine; it's a precious opportunity for self-reflection as you immerse yourself in the rhythm and flow of each movement.

Embrace the stretches, relish the experience, and take pride in waking up every morning empowered by this straightforward yet impactful routine. Throughout the pages of this book, I've shared numerous captivating stories that address all the common questions about engaging with wall Pilates. From the fundamental concepts down to the daily stretches and exercises, we've covered it all. You now have insights on how to dress, set up your personal space at home, what to acquire, and how to fuel your body with better food choices. Armed with the knowledge that wall Pilates provides a secure, controlled, and effective approach to alleviating pain, you can confidently anticipate feeling stronger, more flexible, and capable of an enhanced range of motion in both your legs and arms.

As you've grasped, the essence of Pilates lays the foundation for a unique and comprehensive approach to both exercise and overall well-being. Achieving a centered state is vital for core stability, and you've already understood the significance of maintaining control of your movements, focusing on posture, and synchronizing it all with deliberate breathing. When embarking on your daily wall Pilates routine, invite yourself into a gentle state of flow. Above all, remember to infuse some enjoyment into the process and visualize the goals you're working towards during your workout sessions. Importantly, there's no need to feel pressured; being present in the moment and relishing the sensation of each movement is key.

Take a moment to pause and hydrate with some water in between your exercises. Enhance your workout experience by playing your favorite music. Select something soothing or uplifting to infuse an inspirational dimension. Music serves as a powerful motivator during exercise, especially when it aligns with your personal preferences. Consider incorporating music into your morning routine as well; waking up to meditate on your breath while watching the sunrise, accompanied by calming music, can be both motivating and grounding. As you engage in gentle stretching, let soothing music accompany the nourishment of your body. Feel free to expand your exercise routine as you progress, perhaps with a nature walk or a relaxing swim.

While adding activities, stay mindful of your physical limits and consult with a trusted medical professional to ensure your choices align with your health goals. There will be days when your motivation might not be as strong as before. Rather than interpreting it as a signal to give up, acknowledge it as a passing phase and reassure yourself that tomorrow brings a new opportunity for wall Pilates. Motivation naturally fluctuates, and life's challenges may occasionally interfere. The key is not to abandon your commitment entirely. Remind yourself daily of the reasons driving you to embark on this journey, and consider your body as your newfound ally.

Push through, even when feeling low, as engaging in the routine will uplift your spirits and set a positive tone for the day ahead. The challenges of aging can manifest physically during the golden years, prompting us to prioritize feeling great both internally and externally. It's not about aspiring to replicate the super fitness of our twenties; rather, it's about gracefully honoring a body that has faithfully served us for decades. Committing to daily exercise can rejuvenate your vitality, infuse a radiant glow to your skin, and render your muscles and joints supple, flexible, and ready for added activity. Stepping out of your comfort zone may feel daunting at first, but I assure you that the daily gratitude you'll feel for taking that step will far outweigh any initial apprehensions.

Grant yourself and your body the time needed to adapt to the changes you're implementing. Approach this new holistic lifestyle suggested in the pages of this book with patience, kindness, and gentleness. Consistent effort is the cornerstone of wellness, far superior to a sedentary existence. When faced with challenges, resist the urge to give up; instead, take that initial step towards fortifying and nourishing your body. With each subsequent step on your wall Pilates journey, express gratitude for the remarkable life you've lived and continue to live. I have confidence in your capabilities. You've got this. Wishing you well on your wall Pilates journey, and I look forward to hearing your feedback. Keep radiating your light, love, and wisdom in the world.

REFERENCES

Arm Stretches for Seniors and the Elderly – ELDERGYM®. (n.d.). https://
eldergym.com/arm-stretches/

Austrew, A. (2022, March 18). *Balance issues in older adults: How to help
when dizziness strikes*. Care.com Resources. https://www.care.
com/c/balance-issues-in-older-adults/

Bartlett, D. (2018, May 15). *Five Reasons Modification Is Excellent*. Team
Body Project. https://teambodyproject.com/uncategorized/fiv
e-reasons-modification-excellent/

Brown, J. (2023, November 18). *27 Key Benefits of Wall Pilates: Mind
& Body Wellness - Fitt & Strong*. Https://Fittandstrong.com/.
https://fittandstrong.com/benefits-of-wall-pilates/

Cronkleton, E. (2020, May 11). *Balance Exercises for Seniors: 11
Moves to Try*. Healthline. https://www.healthline.com/health/
exercise-fitness/balance-exercises-for-seniors#balance-tips

Blanchfield, T. (2022, September 22). *Want to Feel More Relaxed? Try
These Deep Breathing Techniques*. Verywell Mind. https://www.
verywellmind.com/the-benefits-of-deep-breathing-5208001

Blanchfield, T. (2022b, September 22). *Want to Feel More Relaxed? Try These Deep Breathing Techniques*. Verywell Mind. https://www.verywellmind.com/the-benefits-of-deep-breathing-5208001

Breathing in Pilates: Why It's Important | Pilates Principles | Club Pilates. (n.d.). Blog.clubpilates.com.au. Retrieved January 10, 2024, from https://blog.clubpilates.com.au/blog/pilates/why-breathing-is-important-in-pilates

Concha-Cisternas, Y., Castro-Piñero, J., Leiva-Ordóñez, A. M., Valdés-Badilla, P., Celis-Morales, C., & Guzmán-Muñoz, E. (2023). *Effects of Neuromuscular Training on Physical Performance in Older People: A Systematic Review*. Life, *13*(4), 869. https://doi.org/10.3390/life13040869

Cristol, H. (2021, March 26). *How Posture Changes as You Get Older*. WebMD. https://www.webmd.com/healthy-aging/features/posture-changes-older-adults

Deep Breathing Exercises, Benefits, and How to Breathe Correctly. (2013, January 19). Robins Key. https://www.robinskey.com/10-benefits-of-deep-breathing/

Dodd, K. (2020, February 14). *Seven Key Nutrients for Senior Nutrition*. The Geriatric Dietitian. https://thegeriatricdietitian.com/7-key-nutrients-for-senior-nutrition/

Exercise Can Help Patients With Rheumatic Disease Live Well. (2013, October 1). The Rheumatologist. https://www.the-rheumatologist.org/article/exercise-can-help-patients-with-rheumatic-disease-live-well/

Fard, M. F. (2022, August 15). *How to Use a Mini-Trampoline*. Experience Life. https://experiencelife.lifetime.life/article/how-to-use-a-mini-trampoline/

Fifty Cardio Exercises for Seniors. (2018, October 6). Vive Health. https://www.vivehealth.com/blogs/resources/cardio-exercises-for-seniors

Five Benefits of Exercise for Seniors and Aging Adults. (2016). The Greenfields. https://thegreenfields.org/5-benefits-exercise-seniors-aging-adults/

Freutel, N. (2016, January 13). *Stretching Exercises for Seniors: Improve Mobility.* Healthline. https://www.healthline.com/health/senior-health/stretching-exercises

GCS, D. K. L., PT, DPT. (2023, May 4). *Why Cardio is Important for Seniors.* The Senior Centered PT. https://theseniorcenteredpt.com/cardio/

Goddard, M. (2018, January 22). *Why You're Losing Motivation as You Age – HealthGuidance.* https://www.healthguidance.org/entry/18054/1/why-youre-losing-motivation-as-you-age.html

Grebeniuk, J. M., I. (2022, November 9). *Wall Pilates For Beginners: Your Complete Guide To Get Started.* BetterMe Blog. https://betterme.world/articles/wall-pilates-for-beginners/

Here's What You Doing Wrong & 7 Other Benefits To Breathing Right. (2023, August 29). Greenlivingtribe. https://greenlivingtribe.com/people-dont-breathe-correctly-slows-weight-loss-what-your-doing-wrong-7-benefits-breathing-right/

Hicks, Tony. (2020, October 6). *As You Get Older, You Need to Drink More Water. Here's Why.* Healthline. https://www.healthline.com/health-news/as-you-get-older-you-need-to-drink-more-water-heres-why

Houston, D. (2019, May 9). *The Crown Chakra: Meanings, Properties and Powers - Complete Guide.* CrystalsandJewelry.com. https://meanings.crystalsandjewelry.com/crown-chakra/

How Exercise Can Boost Your Mood. (2020, June 11). UMMS Health. https://health.umms.org/2020/06/11/exercise-mood/

How to Do Standing Knee Raise Exercise with Proper Technique? (n.d.). Simply Fitness. https://www.simplyfitness.com/pages/standing-knee-raise

Manheim, A. (2023, September 28). *How to Breathe the Pilates Way.* Pilates Anytime. https://www.pilatesanytime.com/blog/more/how-to-breathe-the-pilates-way

Mazzo, L. (2023, May 1). *This Wall Pilates Workout Should Be Your New Bare-Minimum Monday" Routine.* Popsugar. https://www.popsugar.com/fitness/wall-pilates-workout-49156526

McCoy, J. (2023, May 3). *13 Mental Strategies to Help You Stick With Your New Exercise Routine.* SELF. https://www.self.com/story/mental-strategies-to-stick-with-exercise-routine

Mental health includes anxiety and depression. (2020). Dietitiansaustralia.org.au. https://dietitiansaustralia.org.au/health-advice/mental-health-including-anxiety-and-depression

Menzies, R. (2019, December 19). *Pilates for stress relief? Yes!* Pilates Anytime. https://www.pilatesanytime.com/blog/restorative/why-you-should-try-pilates-for-stress-relief

Menzies, R. (2021, October 12). *Pilates for Seniors: Benefits, Considerations, and More.* Healthline. https://www.healthline.com/health/fitness/pilates-for-seniors

Mind & Body Connection: Helping Seniors Stay Healthy - California Mobility. (2019, August 14). Californiamobility.com. https://californiamobility.com/mind-and-body-connection-helping-seniors-stay-healthy/

Morero, C. (2022, March 26). *21/90 Rule - How Long Does It Take to Form a Habit?* SaturdayGift. https://www.saturdaygift.com/21-90-rule/

Nast, C. (2019, July 26). *Did you know Pilates was born in prison and inspired by cats?* Vogue India. https://www.vogue.in/wellness/content/history-of-pilates-workout-born-in-prison-and-inspired-by-cats

Nine Facts You Should Know When Personal Training Senior Citizens. (n.d.). ASFA. https://www.americansportandfitness.com/blogs/fitness-blog/9-facts-you-should-know-when-personal-training-senior-citizens

Nunez, K. (2019, May 31). *Seated Row: Muscles Used, Common Mistakes, Modifications.* Healthline. https://www.healthline.com/health/seated-row

Nutrition for Older Adults. (n.d.). Medlineplus.gov. https://medline-plus.gov/nutritionforolderadults.html#:~:text=Good%20nutri-tion%20is%20important%2C%20no%20matter%20what%20your

Ortiz, D. (2018, August 8). *5 Reasons to Avoid Red Meat in the Senior Years [Guide].* Home Care Assistance of Jefferson County. https://www.homecareassistancejeffersonco.com/why-should-seniors-stop-eating-meat/

Pacheco, D., & Cotliar, D. (2021, January 22). *Caffeine & sleep problems.* Sleep Foundation. https://www.sleepfoundation.org/nutrition/caffeine-and-sleep

Pilates and Knee Pain: Understanding the Causes and Solutions. (2024, January 2). A4 Fitness. https://www.a4fitness.com/why-does-pilates-hurt-my-knees/

Pilates Safety: Minimizing Risks and Preventing Injuries. (2023, May 25). The Secrets of Pilates. https://pilatesecrets.com/can-you-injure-yourself-doing-pilates/

Pilates Tips and Modifications for Wrist Pain. (n.d.). Pilates Anytime. Retrieved January 16, 2024, from https://www.pilatesanytime.com/blog/restorative/pilates-tips-and-modifications-for-wrist-pain

Senior Tip. (2019, June 19). https://ptandme.com/blog/senior-tip-how-physical-exercise-benefits-mental-health/

Shrader, J. (2021, July 29). *A Deep-Breathing Exercise That Reduces Anxiety | Psychology Today.* Www.psychologytoday.com. https://www.psychologytoday.com/us/blog/crazy-life/202107/deep-breathing-exercise-actually-reduces-anxiety

Sleep disorders in older adults: MedlinePlus Medical Encyclopedia. (2017). MedlinePlus. https://medlineplus.gov/ency/article/000064.htm

Smith, R. (2018, May 16). *Pilates Principles - The 6 guiding principles of Pilates.* Complete Pilates. https://complete-pilates.co.uk/pilates-principles/

Ten Best Yoga Poses For Balancing The Throat Chakra. (2023, January 4). Everything Yoga Retreat. https://www.everythingyogaretreat.com/yoga-poses-throat-chakra/

Here's What You Doing Wrong & 7 Other Benefits To Breathing Right. (2023, August 29). Greenlivingtribe. https://greenlivingtribe.com/people-dont-breathe-correctly-slows-weight-loss-what-your-doing-wrong-7-benefits-breathing-right/

How Exercise Can Boost Your Mood. (2020, June 11). UMMS Health. https://health.umms.org/2020/06/11/exercise-mood/

How to Do Standing Knee Raise Exercise with Proper Technique? (n.d.). Simply Fitness. https://www.simplyfitness.com/pages/standing-knee-raise

Smith, A. (2022, May 20). *Top 5 Steps to Creating a Successful Exercise Program | Orlando, FL.* Cflaccidentinjury.com. https://cflaccidentinjury.com/top-5-steps-to-creating-a-successful-exercise-program/

Suni, E. (2023, September 8). *What Is Circadian Rhythm?*

Sleep Foundation. https://www.sleepfoundation.org/circadian-rhythm

Ten Best Yoga Poses For Balancing The Throat Chakra. (2023, January 4). Everything Yoga Retreat. https://www.everythingyogaretreat.com/yoga-poses-throat-chakra/

Tweed, K. (2022, August 7). *6 Myths About Exercise and Aging.* WebMD. https://www.webmd.com/fitness-exercise/exercise-and-aging-myths

Ullrich, P. (2019). *Low Back Pain in Older Adults.* Spine-Health. https://www.spine-health.com/conditions/lower-back-pain/low-back-pain-older-adults

Venkat, S. R. (2022, August 8). *What to Know About Core Exercises for Seniors?* WebMD. https://www.webmd.com/fitness-exercise/what-to-know-about-core-exercises-for-seniors

Walsh, G. (2023, September 17). *I tried indoor cycling for a month - and these are the benefits I experienced.* Woman and Home Magazine. https://www.womanandhome.com/health-wellbeing/benefits-of-indoor-cycling/

What To Do If You Have Neck Pain In Pilates. (2023, November 17). Pilatesology. https://pilatesology.com/2023/11/what-to-do-if-yo u-have-neck-pain-in-pilates/

Woods, L. (2020, June 4). *Benefits of Leg Workouts, or Why You Shouldn't Skip Your Leg Day.* BetterMe Blog. https://betterme.world/ articles/benefits-of-leg-workouts/

Working out boosts brain health. (2020, March 4). Apa.org; American Psychological Association. https://www.apa.org/topics/exercise-fitness/stress

Dear Reader,

As you turn the last page of "Wall Pilates for Seniors Made Easy," we hope you feel invigorated and inspired, equipped with the tools to enhance your functional strength, stability, and vitality. This 28-day guide is crafted to help you reclaim the energy and mobility of your younger years, even as you navigate the complexities of aging.

Now, we invite you to share your journey with others. Your review can light the way for many who are just starting or contemplating their path to better health. It's not merely about sharing your success; it's about inspiring a community of seniors to embrace a life of independence and joy.

Your Review Matters

Your insights are invaluable. They provide real-life context to the effectiveness of the exercises, the clarity of the illustrations, and the overall impact of the program on your daily life. You're not just offering feedback; you're offering hope and encouragement to someone who may be hesitating to take the first step.

How to Leave a Review

1. Visit the website where you purchased your book.
2. Navigate to the "Wall Pilates for Seniors Made Easy" page.
3. Click on 'Customer Reviews' then select 'Write a Review.'

4. Share your thoughts about the book. What improvements have you noticed in your own life? Which exercises have become your favorites? How has the book made your everyday activities easier?

You don't need to write a lengthy review—just a few heartfelt sentences can greatly influence someone else's journey towards better health.

Alternatively, if you're viewing this digitally, you might see a QR Code below. Simply scan it with your camera to be taken directly to the review page.

Your voice has the power to motivate, inspire, and perhaps even transform someone's life. Thank you for taking the time to spread positivity and support through your words.

With much gratitude for your help,
Brenda ten Bosch

Made in the USA
Monee, IL
07 November 2024

69598501R00105